AYURVEDA

OR THE

HINDU SYSTEM OF MEDICAL SCIENCE

AYURVEDA

OR THE

HINDU SYSTEM OF MEDICAL SCIENCE

BY

MANMATHANATH DATTA

GYAN

Published by

Gyan Publishing House
5, Ansari Road
Daryaganj, New Delhi-110002
Phone: 011-47034999, 9811692060
E-mail: books@gyanbooks.com

Distribution Network
gyanbooks.com
India, USA, Canada, UK, Australia

ISBN: 978-93-6920-533-2 (HB)
First Published, 1899

2nd Impression 2025

Printed at: Gyan Press, Delhi.

AYURVEDA OR THE HINDU SYSTEM OF MEDICAL SCIENCE
Author: MANMATHANATH DATTA

AYURVEDA.

AYURVEDA

OR THE

HINDU SYSTEM OF MEDICAL SCIENCE

PUBLISHED BY

THE SOCIETY FOR THE RESUSCITATION OF

INDIAN LITERATURE.

Calcutta:

PRINTED BY H. C. DASS,

THE ELYSIUM PRESS, 65/2 BEADON STREET.

1899.

PREFACE.

A POPULAR History of Hindu Medicine is a desideratum in English Literature ;—and yet the growing spirit of the age calls for a systematic arrangement of the subject. This miniature History of Hindu *Ayur-Veda* is the growth of the times. Amidst the mass of writings scattered in the pages of forgotten works on classical Hind, this little book will, it is hoped, serve as beacons in directing the foot-steps of the rising generation, and tend to inspire them with zeal to pursue their course of investigation in the realms of antiquity, and stimulate them to fulfil the heritage of the intellectual glory of their sires worthy of the tradition of their race.

It now remains to add that the materials of this sketch were mostly gleaned from the monumental work of Dr. Thomas A. Wise, to the genius of whose pen the world is indebted for a comprehensive *Review of the History of Medicine*.

CONTENTS.

—:o:—

Subject.	Page.
Antiquity of the Hindu Medical System ...	1
Mythical Account of the Antiquity of Ayur-Veda	5
Historical Account of the Antiquity of Ayur-Veda	10
Hindu Medical Works and their Authors ...	22
Synopsis of the Leading Medical Works (Atreya Samhita)	29
Analysis of Charaka	33
Sushruta	39
The Rank of the Hindu Physicians	43
The Duty of the Physician and his Attendants	44
The Physician's fees	51
Hindu Physiology: Growth of the Human Body	53
The Three Period of a Man's Life	61
Structure of the Body	62
Hindu Materia Medica	73
Hindu Pharmacy	80
Hindu Hygiene	112
Hindu Surgery	119

AYURVEDA

OR THE

HINDU SYSTEM OF MEDICAL SCIENCE.

CHAPTER I.

THE ANTIQUITY OF THE HINDU MEDICAL SYSTEM.

After an apathy of ages, the medical system of the Rishis has again attracted the admiration of the world. Like various other departments of science and literature, the Hindu medical system claims to be the first of its kind in the world and has lent much towards the advancement of the medical systems of other countries. Truly does Dr. Wise remark, "Asia can munificently give, but it does not need to borrow: its ideas and phantasies are as exhuberant as its vegetation." This remark is not only applicable to the philosophy, theology and other departments of Aryan thought, but is equally so to their medical system. It is the growth of their own soil, and their medicines are the products of their own mart.

If we carefully study our own literature, we shall find that our medical system was introduced early in the Vedic age. Although it did not then assume the shape of a regular scientific system, yet we can infer the existence of medical practice from various passages in Vedic poetry. There are several hymns in which are recorded the hygenic properties of water, air and vegetables. The following hymn supports our assertion.

"I invoke the divine waters in which our cattle drink. Ambrosia is in the waters: in the waters are medicinal herbs."

In the pantheon of the Rigveda, Soma is the presiding deity of medicinal herbs. Rishi Medathiti addressed a hymn to him which will give a very clear idea as to the earliest reference to medicinal herbs. The hymn runs thus :—

"Soma has declared to me all medicaments as well as Agni, the benefactor of the universe are in the waters ; waters contain all healing herbs.

Waters bring to perfection all diseases dispensing medicaments for (the good of) my body, that I may long behold the sun."

The twin gods Aswinis have always been described as the physicians of the gods. They are the twin children of the sun and many of their marvellous cures are recorded in the Rigveda. There is a hymn by the Rishi Kakshivat in which they are praised for curing blindness and deafness. The hymn is :

"Hear the song of the stumbling blind man, for verily, Aswinis, I glorify you for recovering my eyes through you, who are protectors of good works.

Kanwa obtained his eye-sight from them and the son of Nrishada his hearing, as the following hymn says :

"You gave relief to the imprisoned Atri. Solicitous of worthy praise, you gave sight to Kanwa blinded by darkness."

In another hymn by Gristamada, we find Rudra invoked as the bestower of health.

"Nursed by the sanitory vegetables which are bestowed by thee, may I live a hundred winters: extirpate my enemies, my exceeding sin and my manifold infirmities.

Let us not provoke thee, Rudra, to wrath by our imperfect adorations; invigorate our sons by the medicinal plants. For I hear that thou art a chief physician among physicians."

In various other subsequent verses, Rudra has been invoked for healing herbs and medicaments. That there were medical practitioners in the Vedic period, is also proved by the following verse of the Rigveda translated by Dr. Muir:

"I am a poet, my father is a doctor and mother a grinder of corn. With our different views, seeking to get gain, we run after our respective objects."

From what we have said before, it is evident that during the Vedic period medicinal herbs were known to the ancient Hindus and their use was oftentimes resorted to for the cure of various ailments. But it did not become a regular science till the Puranic age. To Hindus, so important was the knowledge of medicine, that it is said to have been revealed by Brahmā and practised by Siva, Indra, Surya and the two Ashwinis.

CHAPTER II.

THE MYTHICAL ACCOUNT OF THE ANTIQUITY OF AYURVEDA.

The mythological account of the Hindus traces the origin of *Ayurvedâ*, their medical science, in the beginning of the *Kali yuga*, when *Brahmâ*, taking compassion on man's weak, degenerate and suffering state, produced the *Upaveda* or commentary on the sacred *Vedas*, which consists of four treatises (1) the *Dharmashâstra*, the science of law (2) *Dhanurveda*, the science of the bow, (3) *Gandharva Veda*, the science of music, (4) *Ayurveda* the science of life. Thus a systematic treatise on medical science is given by *Brahmâ* to mankind to teach them properly the manner of living in the world by preventing and curing diseases. This sacred medical work of the Hindus resembles in form and style the fourth sacred *Veda* mamely the *Atharvan.* It describes the means of keeping health, the causes of diseases and the ways of curing them. The original work was divided into eight sections. They are :—

(1). *Salya* or surgery; it deals with the method of removing external substances such as grass, wood, stones &c. accidently getting into the body: explains the method of removing dead child from the mother's womb, of healing wounds and using various surgical instruments in operations.

(2). *Salakya*; it deals with the description and treatment of the external and organic diseases of the eyes, ears, mouth and nose &c.

(3). *Kâya Chikitsâ* or an account of the diseases affecting the whole body as fevers, consumption, mania, epilepsy, leprosy, diabetes and other diseases.

(4). *Bhuta Vidyâ* or the means of restoring the deranged faculties of the mind on account of a man's being possessed by devils.

(5) *Kaumarabhritya* or the treatment of infantile diseases.

(6). *Agada* or the administration of poisons and their antedotes.

(7). *Rasâyana* or an account of the medicines which cure all diseases, restore general health and youth.

(8). *Bâjikarana* or the means of restoring the manhood and increasing the human race.

Thus we see that *Ayurdeva* is the first systemetic work on Hindu medicine which was revealed by Brahmā who first instructed the patriarch Daksha. He wrote a book named *Chikitsâ-darshana* and communicated the medical science to the two Ashwinis or off-spring of the sun. Others say that Brahmā communicated the Ayurveda to Surya. The Ashwinis were the medical attendants of the gods and authors of several treatises on medicine one of which was named *Chikitsa-ratnatantra.* As the gods were ever youthful and healthy suffering from no diseases they stood in no need of a physician. The

Ashwinis however performed many surgical operations for the gods. Being cured of his paralytic arm by the Ashwinis Indra learnt Ayurveda from them.

Thus it is evident that for a considerable time the knowledge of *Ayurveda* was confined amongst the gods. Sometime after this, however, with the prevalence of wickedness and iniquity, mankind began to suffer from various' diseases. Grieved at this, the sages *Varadwàja* and *Atreya* convened a meeting of the *Munis* in the Himalaya mountains. According to the account in Charaka there were present the sages Angira, Jamadagni, Vasistha, Kasyapa, Bhrigu. Atreya, Gautama, Sankhya, Pulastya, Narada, Asita, Bamdeva, Markandeya, Aswanayana, Parikshita, Bhikshuratreya, Bharadwaja, Kapinjala, Vishwāmitra, Aswaranya, Bhargava, Chayabana, Abhijit, Gargya, Sandilya, Kaundilya, Abarkshi, Devala, Galava, Saukritya, Vaijavapaya, Kusika, Vadarayna, Kaikasaey, Dhauma, Marichi, Kasyapa, Sarakarakshya, Hiranakshya, Lokakshya, Paingi, Saunaka, Sakuneya, Gautamayani and others.

After some deliberations they all arrived at the conclusion that the only means of saving humanity from such a disaster was to send one of their number to the thousand-eyed deity Indra and to obtain from him the knowledge of medicine. Varadwāja was selected. The sage went to the king of gods and returned with the knowledge of Ayurveda. He related to the Rishis the precepts that he had learnt from Indra. They consisted of (1) *Samana* or the general character of everything, (2) *Visesa* or classification, (3) *Dravya* or elements, (4) *Guna* or qualities, (5) *Karma* or actions, (6) *Sanyoga* or combination. Of those Rishis Atreya communicated his knowledge of medicine to his numerous pupils.

Then again after the deluge when the Vedas were lost the gods and demons churned the ocean for finding out the water of immortality. When the ocean was churned many precious gifts or *ratnas* came out. Among them was Dhanwantari the physician or holy sage who came out with water of life or *Amrita*. He was a pupil of

Indra in Ayurveda and practised medicine in heaven. Seeing the miseries and diseases of mankind he came down on earth to instruct them in the science of life. He afterwards became the king of Kasi and performed many celebrated cures. Witnessing the miserable condition of mankind the Rishis sent a deputation to Divadasa or Dhanwantari requesting him to teach them the science of life. This deputation consiststed of Oupadhnuba, Baiturana, Aurabhra, Karabirja, Goupura, Rukeeta and Susruta who followed the king to retirement. Of them Susruta was selected to abridge theAyurveda.

CHAPTER III.

HISTORICAL ACCOUNT OF THE ANTIQUITY OF AYURVEDA.

FOR years it has been a prevailing belief in Europe that she borrowed her medical Science from Greece. It is an undeniable truth that the civilization of the western world has drawn its inspiration from Greece. In every department of literature and art we find the traces of Greek origin. As the the modern philosophy is indebted to Greece for its first ideas, so is the medical Science of the west is indebted to her for its origin. It has again been proved by ancient scholars of the west, that Greece also obtained her medical science from Egypt and Arabia.

Hitherto facts regarding the ancient history of medicine have been sought for in Greece, and Rome and any system that did not trace its origin from either of these sources was repudiated. This belief was owing to the prevailing ignorance of the western scholars regarding history of India and other Eastern countries. But during the last half of the present century great progress has been made in the knowledge of the Asiatic empires by the learned labours of such eminent scholars as Sir William Jones and Professor Wilson. The unfolding of the learning of the Egyptians, the exhumation of the Assyrian and Babylonian monuments, the study of the sacred books of India have brought to light a considerable amount of new, but momentous facts which have clearly proved that for the first conception of the medical science the whole world is indebted to the Rishis of India. We will attempt to prove this statement in the following pages from historical evidences.

We need not attempt to prove that Greece is the mother of the medical Science of the west, for it is a fact of history that has been proved beyond any shadow of doubt. The following facts, taken from the ancient history of Greece will conclusively prove that Greece is indebted elsewhere for her medical science.

Artaxarxes sent an invitation to the great Hippocrates to come over to his court on the occasion of the ravages of the plague. But this great physician could not comply with the request of the king as his services were required in his own country, then suffering under the same fell disease.

Again in B. C. 405 Ctesias, a descendant of Asclepiades was taken prisoner. He healed the wound of king Artaterxes Mnemon and was kept there as his physician. He served in this capacity for seventeen years and went several times to Greece as an ambassador. He wrote several historical works one of which was on India.

Darius Hystaspes conquered India about B.C. 530 and it was the richest of his twenty satrapies. Two centuries afterwards Alexander destroyed the Persian Empire and on his approaching India Taxiles conciliated the Greek envoy by presents saying :—" I shall send to the great conqueror your master, my beautiful daughter, a goblet of ruby ; a philosopher of great knowledge of the sciences, and a physician who has such skill that he can restore the dead." This shows that India had good and skillful physicians at the time when Alexander conquered her.

Nearchus (*Apud* Arrian) says that " the Greek physicians found no remedy againgst the bite of snakes; but the Indians cured those who happened to incur that misforture." Accordingly he issued an edict ordering that all persons, bitten by snakes, should be sent to his tent where the Indian physicians would cure—and so of many other incurable diseases.

Egypt was the first country that profitted much by eastern learning which they communicated to the western branch of the family of man inhabiting the shores of Hellespont and the Ægean sea. Many Sanskrit words appear in Greek authors: this proves the early connection between the two countries. Besides many medicines produced in India were used by early Greeks.

Though the popular belief is that the various medical systems of Europe were derived from the family of Hippocrates and that with some hints from the Egyptians the Greeks first originated the medical science and art of Europe, still, from recent investigations it has been conclusively proved that they really obtained it from the Hindus, whose medical knowledge the Egyptian priesthood communicated to the philosophers of Greece. It was Hippocrates who first compiled a systematic work on medicine which was the first text book for the Western world. It was not possible for one man, with the greatest possible industry, to have compiled such a voluminous record and so the natural inference is that Hippocrates must have taken advantage of the labours of his predecessors and have obtained assistance from elsewhere.

It is said that besides taking advantage of the recorded experience of his predecessors this great man travelled in many countries to collect information. Galen mentions that Hippocrates was at Smyrna in Asia Minor. Mercurial proved that he travelled in Sybia, in Africa and Scythia in Asia. What could have induced him to visit this distant country except his information regarding the medical knowledge of the people there?

That Hippocrates derived assistance from the Hindus is evident from the number of Indian, plants imported from there to Greece, mentioned in his Materia Medica and used for their well-known properties by the Greeks, such as Sessamum Indicum-Lin; hyperanthera morunga, &c.

The Greek physician Actuarius speaks of the Hindu medicine *tryphala.* Though he does not mention it as a Hindu medicine he speaks of the peculiar products of India of which it is compesed by their Sanskrit name Myrobalans. Another physician, by name Ætius, a native of Amida, in Mesopotamia, who studied at Alexandria about the end of the fifth century, not only speaks of the Myrobalans, but mentions it as the proper remedy for elephantisis, a disease very common in India.

From the internal evidence it is clear that Hippocrates' works were mere compilations derived partly from other nations who were more advanced than the Greeks in the healing art. The Hindu surgeons were most clever in Surgery and they used to perform most difficult operations as Cæsarian section, embryotomy, lithotomy, &c. Amongst the western authors Celsus gives an account of the last operation and in his work he mentions the names of the two Egyptian lithotomists. It is evident from this that he may have derived his knowledge of Surgery from

Egypt than from Persia and Arabia the medical men of which countries did not attend much to Surgery. They were on the other hand so much prejudiced against the operation of lithotomy that even to witness it was considered disreputable by their most able surgical writer Avenzoar.

It was the practice with Hyppocrates that he used to take an oath from his pupils not to perform an operation of lithotomy, which, was left to men who were special practitioners of this operation." From this it is clear that he acquired his surgieal knowledge from some other nation than the Persians and Arabians—and this nation was none but the Hindus.

We have thus shown that Greece borrowed her medical science from elsewhere and that the study of medicine was successfully pursued for many centuries in India before it could attain to that stage in which Alexander found it in the fourth century B.C. If we can prove that Egypt, China, Persia, and Arabia obtained their knowledge of medicine from India, it will then be established beyond any doubt that the Aryan Rishis were the first who bequeathed to the humanity the healing art.

Civilization, in China and Egypt, is of a very enduring character and it is probable that their knowledge of arts and science is earlier than that of any other nation. The recorded history however of China does not go further back than the reign of Chi-Hoang-te Schiboany who lived 240 years before the birth of Christ. The ancient Chinese records clearly prove that there existed intimate intercourse between China and India before the Christian ere by means of travellers and ambassadors. At a very early period Buddhist Monks carried to China treatises on Hindu medicine and translated them. It is also seen that science of medicine was systematically introduced in China by Chung-ke only about A. D. 229.

The Egyptians were better known to the Europeans than the Chinese; the Egyptians acquired their rudiments of learning from the East. Herodotus, Diogenes, Laertius and Plutarch learnt from here what they taught in Greece. The records found in the temples of Abydos and Sais prove that the Egyptians obtained their religious systems from India. They directly obtained their religion from Ethiopia and Miroe which countries again obtained it from India. This is held by such eminent men as Herodotus, Plato, Solon, Pythagorus and Philostratus. This is equally proved by the fact that both the systems proceeded from the monotheistic principles and ultimately degenerated into polytheism. Again the Hindu *Puranas* hold that a mission was sent to Ethiopia and Egypt which conveyed their sacred Vedas. The Brahmins also assert that Pythagorus and Zerdusht were their disciples.

Again in the Shah Nama Ferdusi states that Kykasos, one of the kings, was a Brahmin. Sheikh Abu Soliman, the logician, states that his teacher Ibu Ady who died at Bagdad, A. D. 974, assured him that the Hindus possessed more sublime ideas regarding religion and philosophy.

More modern historical facts also prove that Greece, Arabia, Persia, all profitted greatly by the learning of the Hindu physicians.

When the Emperor Valirian was taken a captive by Sapor I. in A. D. 262, Sapor II. married the daughter of the Emperor Aurilian and used to encourage much the learned men of the East. Many Greek philosophers and physicians used to resort to his court which became celebrated as the medical school where Rhazes, and Haly Abbas were educated. The Hindu medical work Charaka is mentioned in the works of Rhazes and Sarapion. It has also been proved that the Charaka and Susruta were translated and studied by the Arabians in the day of Harul-al-Rashid and Mansur A. D. 773. Al-Mansur caused translations to be made from the Sanskrit of medical scientific works among which are particularly mentioned "a tract upon poisons" by Shanak (meaning Charak; and a treatise on Meteria medica by Shashrud meaning Sushrutta.

Baron de Sacy also mentions that the Fables of Pilpay were first translated from Sanskrit in the sixth century by the physician

Barzouyeh at the command of Al Mansur who removed the seat of the Arab Government from Damuscus to Bagdad, and who had twice gone to India for procuring Indian medical works and herbs at the command of the Persian king Neserwan.

Another well-known physician who followed Rhazes was Avicenna, otherwise called Sheikh Reyes or the prince of physicians. He was born in Bokhara. Avicenna was well known for his acquirements even at an early age. In treating of leeches Avicienna begins as "what the Indian says" and gives exactly the very words of Shshruta describing the six poisonous leeches.

In the reign of Harul-al-Rashid not only the Hindu medical works were valued but the Hindu physicians actually lived at his court. Ibu Osaiba states that Manka was an emineut Hindu physician well read in Sanskrit literature. He made a journey from India to Iraca, cured the Khalif of an illness and translated a work on poison by Charaka from Sanskrit into Persian. Ibu Osaiba mentions the name of another Hindu physician, Saleh who lived at the court of Harun-al Rashid. He travelled to Egypt and Palestine, died and was burried in Egypt.

These historical facts, culled from the records of other nations, conclusively prove that India has given the medical science to the world. The humanity should be grateful to the Aryan Rishis for the healing Art, and their Indian Medical Science is as old as their Veda, which we have already proved from mythical accounts.

CHAPTER IV.

HINDU MEDICAL WORKS AND THEIR AUTHORS.

THE Ayurveda is considered as the most ancient and authoritative work on the Hindu system of medical science. But this work is not to be seen now and only fragments of the manuscripts are procurable. Of the Puranas only the Agnipurana gives an account of the nature of medicines and diseases.

The following works and authors are mentioned in the great epic poem Mahabharata :—

1. Atreya Sanhita by Atreya.
2. Charak by Agnivesa and Charak.
3. Bhilatantra by Bhila.
4. Jatukarnatantra by Jatukarna.
5. Parasara Sanhita by Parasara.
6. Harita Sanhita by Harita.
7. Karparitantra by Karpari.
8. Shusruta by Dhanwantari and Shusruta.

Of these works, the third, fourth, fifth and seventh are not procurable. These works were compiled by different sages at different periods after the plan of the original Ayurveda. The oldest existing work on medicine is the Atreya Sanhita ascribed to a son of the Vedic Saint Atri. The most authoritative works, now held in highest esteem by the Hindu physicians, are the Charak and Shusruta. They are in fact the commentaries on the original Ayurveda embodying the compendium of that voluminous work.

Is it not at all possible to give an idea of

the exact date of the composition of these two great medical treatises. Charak ranks next in antiquity to the Atreya Sanhita. And although the Shusruta is considered as the standard work of ancient Hindu medicine Charak Sanhita is a far more interesting work. Charaka was a person of great culture and intellect and prepared his work for the general guidance of the humanity in the ways of life and health. He himself states in his work that at first the material of his great work was communicated by the Rishi Atreya and Agnivesa. From the latter Charak received his instructions, who condensed the original work where it was too prolix for the easy and ready reference of mankind. The result of Charak's labour was however, very voluminous and consisted of one hundred and twenty chapters in eight divisions. It is arranged in the form of dialouges or lectures between the master and the pupil on various practical and important subjeets for the benefit of mankind. The pupil asks questions like the following and the teacher answers them. The pupil asks "what is the soul? How is it produced? Is it intelligent or ignorant? Is it eternal or destructible? Whence does the soul proceed? What is the proof of its existence? What is the disease and how the practioners prevent it?" Thus in this way Charaka has introduced in his great work various subjects relating to the soul, matter, mind and body. In this work simple medicines are employed often in combination. These ingredients were however increased in number by his followers.

Shusruta is reported to have lived later than Charaka. Mythology describes him as the son of Vishwamitra a contemporary of Rama. He was instructed by Dhanwantari in medical science. After Charaka his book is the oldest work on Hindu medicine. It was thus prepared. Dhanwantari asked his pupils on what he would lecture first. They wanted him to lecture on surgery first because it afforded immediate relief. The lectures of Dhanwantari were subsequently arranged by Shusruta after the plan of the original Ayurveda.

The Charaka and Shusruta are thus the

ground work of the medical system of the Hindus, upon which the recent writers have drawn for insperation. Charaka is superior to Sushruta in the acuracy of description, in the classification of diseases and the general plan of treatment, whereas Sushruta excels him in anatomical descriptions and the treatment of surgical diseases. He surpassed Charaka in Salya or the art of extracting extraneous substances and Salakya or the treatment of external organs. On the authority of Dhanwantari he declares that Salya is "the first or the best of the medical sciences; less liable than any other to the fallacy of conjectural and inferential practice; pure in itself; perpetual in its applicability; the worthy produce of heaven and certain of fame." And although he pays the greatest attention to surgery he also discusses the treatment of general diseases and management of women. He also describes many mechanical modes of giving immediate relief in an illness. He speaks of one hundred and one surgical implements but always says that "the first, best and the most important is hand." He also enumerates twenty surgical instruments made of metal.

Sushruta spoke highly of dissection as necessary for the attainment of competent medical knowledge. He says that "the teacher shall seek to perfect his pupil by the application of all expedients which he may think calculated to effect his proficiency."

Besides these two most sacred and authoritative medical works of the Hindus there are many important professional commentaries on different medical subjects. Of them the two deserve most attention. *Bhagbhata* compiled a treatise called *Ashtángahridaya.* This was mainly compiled from Charaka and Sushruta. The plan and treatment of the subject is almost the same and it is written in a clear and simple style. Another celebrated medical work compiled three hundred years ago is *Bhávaprakásha.* The author made selections of most important subjects from various works and named the compilation after him. Many obscurities of ancient medical works the author has explained by his most beautiful and lucid arrangement.

This work was evidently intended for practitioners and is an admirable account of all the practical parts of the Hindu medical science.

The following is a list, as given in Dr. Wise's learned work, of the principal medical works which are now seen in India. They were all compiled from Charaka and Sushruta. They are arranged in order of date :— Aupadhanaha and Auravhra wrote works on surgery ; Todrananda, Chakradatta, Pracharaратnavali and Sarangadhara wrote on the system of medicine ; Rajanirghanta prepared a Materia Medica to which Dravyaguna added a commentary ; Madhava Nidana a work on Nosology ; Bangajaratnavali is a system of Pharmacy ; Rasa-Ratnākara is a treatise on Metalic preparations ; and Rashendrachintāmani, Rasendrakalpadruma, and Madhumati are works on Hindu medical system.

CHAPTER V.

SYNOPSIS OF THE LEADING MEDICAL WORKS.

ATREYA SAMHITA.

THIS is the oldest existing work on the Hindu medical system written by a son of the Vedic Rishi Atri.

Chapters 1—3 may be considered as a general introduction.

Chapter 1 relates the meeting of Atreya with some of his pupils on the Northern face of the Himalaya. Harita one of those pupils asks questions on the origin and treatment of disease. Atreya explains that the Ayur-Veda, meaning medical science, could not be fully communicated within the limits of human life, and that his pupils must therefore content themselves with a brief account of the smallest of his own compositions which is comprised within 1,500 Slokas.

Chapter 2 shows the general division of his work into six books and gives their names. In conclusion it states the eight constituent parts of the Ayur-Veda.

Chapter 3 classifies diseases, as 1st curable 2nd incurable, 3rd curable by charms; scarcely possible to cure. This chapter also distinguishes the patients to whom physicians must attend and on what terms and signifies to what persons they must refuse assistance.

Chapter 4 treats on the physical influence of soil and season, on age and temper and on the influence of the winds.

Chapter 5 enumerates the six tastes; as sweet, astringent, bitter, sour, salt and pungent and enumerates the influence of each on the human body.

Chapter 6 treats of the medical qualities of different kinds of water: as the water of the Ganges which comes from heaven, water which comes from the sea: water which comes from clouds in general and water which comes from thunder, clouds, snow or ice. This chapter concludes with prescriptions for the use of hot water and cold water in specified diseases.

Chapter 7 discusses the physical and

medical properties of milk:—distinguishing the milk of kine, goats, ewes, buffaloes, camels, women. It states the cases in which the drinking of milk of either kind is beneficient; and concludes by discoursing on the medical properties of butter-milk.

Chapter 8 continues the subject.

Chapter 9 treats on the medical qualities of sugar-cane and of preparations from it.

Chapter 10 on sour gruel.

Chapters 11 and 12 of infusions prepared from rice, barley and other grains.

Chapter 13 on oils prepared from Til, flax, the castor-oil, plant and others.

Chapters 14, 15, 16 also treat on the medical properties of rice and various kinds of grain.

Chapter 17 discuses four kinds of Potherbs, according to their leaves, flowers, fruits and bulbons-roots.

Chapter 18 is on sweet fruits as mangoes, rose-apples, pomegranates, myrobalans, citrons, grapes and the fruits of carisoa-corrianders and of the mimusops eleugi.

Chapter 19 treats on four kinds of spirituous liquor, as made from molasses, honey, meal and nogweed.

Chapter 20 describes animals as hoofed or horned ,beasts of prey, birds, fishes, snakes living in the water or in arid tracts. Many species are given under each division and the medical properties of their flesh are described.

Chapter 21 gives dietitical rules and prescriptions and discusses the properties of food prepared from various combinations of the materials previously described.

The second main division of Atreya's works called Arishtaka consists of eight chapters.

Chapter 1 treats on the moral causes of diseases. All diseases are said to spring for men's actions. All resemble hell, the curable as well as the incurable. And to some crimes fantastic punishments are assigned, as if a man kills a Brahmin he will be afflicted with jaundice, one who kills a king with consumption. Chapter 2 is on dreams.

The subject of the six remaining chapters appears to be lucky and unlucky symptoms and fore-bodings. The third division of this work called Chikitsā which means, as we observed, medical treatment. This portion treats of diseases in detail. It appears to display much accurate observation, which can only be glanced at in these pages. Intermittent fevers are distinguished as of four kinds returning at an interval of one day, three days, four days or at some long intervals.

CHAPTER VI.

ANALYSIS OF CHARAKA.

The first division of Charaka's Sanhitā is called Slokasthāna. It consists of thirty chapters. Chapter I. relates the origin of the work, and gives a brief summary. Chapters 2, 3, and 4 treat on medical plants and their properties. Chapters 5—7 on matters of diet. Chapter 8 on the senses and on the elements with which the senses correspond. Chapters 9 and 10 on the qualities which a physician must possess, and also on the qualities which are indispensable to his medicaments. Chapters 11 and 12 show the means by which long life may be secured and adverse influences counteracted. Chapter 13 treats on fat and on the diseases thence arising. Chapter 14 on perspiration and how it may be produced. Chapter 15 on medical instruments and appliances. Chapter 16 on the presents which a physician should receive. Chapter 17 gives a general enumeration of diseases and their symptoms. Chapter 18 treats on three descriptions of swellings. Chapters 19 and 20 give further enumerations of the diseases and their causes. Chapter 21 is on the eight defects of the constitution, and their influence on health. Chapter 22 on fasting, on getting fat, on sweating &c. Chapter 23 on diseses arising from gourmandising. Chapter 24 on the blood and its affections. Chapter 25 on purusha, which means the soul. Chapter 26 on the 6 flavours *rashas* (sweet, salt, pungent &c.) and effects of these on the body. Chapters 27 and 28 on the effects of different kinds of food and beverage. Chapter 29 on the vital organs. Chapter 30 on the heart. This division concludes with a general eulogy on the Aur-Veda.

The second division of Charaka's work is named *Nidânasthâna*, and treats in eight chapters on the symptoms of certain diseases, as 1 Fever. 2. Plethora. 3. Gulma or enlargement of spleen 4. Twenty varities of urinary disease. 5. Seven kinds of Leprosy 6. Four varieties of Sosha or consumption. 7. Five descriptions of mania. 8. Four kinds of epilepsy.

The third division, called *Vimânasthâna*, likewise consists of eight chapters. Chapter 1 shows the actions of flavour and substance on the body. Chapter 2 the three stages of digestion. Chapter 3 the causes of diseases (climatic and religious). Chapter 4 gives three kinds of diagnosis. Chapter 5 treats on some of the constituent parts of the body. Chapter 6 gives a general description of diseeases (curable and incurable, mental and bodily, organic and accidental &c.) Chapter 7 gives a general classification of patients.

Chapter 8 treats on the modes of studying, medicine, on the manner in which a student of medicine should behave, and how one physician should conduct an argument with another physician. &c.

The fourth division bears the name of Sarirasthāna, and this also contains eight chapters treating on the following subjects. Chapter 1. purusha, soul and its relation to the body and the organs of sense as explained in Hindu philosophy. Chapters 2 to 4 on the fœtus and its physical and moral development. Chapter 5 on the soul, as a part of the body when born. Chapter 6 on the nature of the human body. Chapter 7 enumerates all its parts and Chapter 8 treats on generation.

The fifth division is called Indriyasthāna and has twelve chapters; 1 on color as indicating health on approaching death. 2 on smells and tastes, which forbode death. 3 on feelings which forbode the same. 4 on other symptoms by which physicians may prognosticate life or death. 5 on dreams as forboding death. 7—10 on other bodily symptoms of the same character. 11—12 on omens and other signs independendent of the body which indicate approaching death.

The sixth division is Chikitsāsthāna. It consists of thirty chapters and the subject is therapeutics. Chapters 1 and 2 treat on elixir of life and their preparation. The subjects of the other chapters are as follows. 3 Fever. 4 Plethora. 5 Enlargement of spleen, gulma. 6 Urinary diseses. 7 Leprosy. 8 Consumption. 9 Mania. 10 Epilepsy. 11 A disease of the chest called Kshata Kshina. 12 Swellings. 13 Enlargement of the abdomen. 14 Piles. 15 Dysentery. 16 Pallor. 17 Hiccough. 18 Catarrah. 19 Diarrhœa. 20 Vomiting. 21 Erysipelas. 22 Thirst. 23 Poisoning 24 Raving. 25 Sores. 26 Deseases affecting the three vital cavities (belly, chest, head). 27 Paralysis of the lower extremities. 28 Flatulency. 29 Gout. 30 Diseases of generative organs.

The seventh division, or Kalpasthāna, has twelve chapters which treat on drugs which cause vomiting and purging and on how to administer such drugs in the treatment of diseases. Six hundred medicines of this chracter are mentioned and classified according to the place they come from and their inherent properties.

The eighth and last division is Sidhisthāna. This also consists of twelve chapters. From 1-8 show in what manner the medicines described in the Kalpasthāna should be introduced into the body by means of syringes and tubes and shows also in what cases emetics and purgatives and enemas should not be used. Chapter 9 treats on diseases caused by internal injuries to either of the vital cavities mentioned above, and of treatment of such cases by enemas and purgatives. The vital organs included in these vital cavities (chest, belly, head) are enumerated as one hundred and seven. Chapters 10—12 are again chiefly occupied with the uses of enemas.

CHAPTER VII.

SUSHRUTA.

This is really a work on Hindu surgery communicated by Dhanwantari to his pupils and arranged by the great Rishi Sushruta. The eight divisions of the original Ayurveda are arranged in the following six books by Sushruta.

1st. *Sutrashthána*—medical doctrine. This book deals with miscellaneous introductory subjects, such as the principles of medicine; the origin of medicine; the selection, management and the instruction of pupils; their faculties; the first principles and elements of the body; the various forms of diseases and accidents and their treatment; the rules for teaching; the duty of practitioners; the selection and use of instruments and of medicines; the influence of weather on health and the practice to be followed after surgical operations. Then follows the description of the diseases of the humours and of surgical diseases; the restoration of defective ears and noses; the removal of extraneous substances getting into the body; the different stages of inflammation with their treatment; the different forms of wounds and ulcers; the description of good and bad diet; of prognosis; the kind of messenger to be employed by the sick; and of diseases produced by the deranged actions of the senses and of incurable diseases. Then come the preparations required for accompanying a king in war, the duty of practitioners, the variety of climates and the different classes of medicines. These subjects are treated of in forty-six chapters.

2nd. *Nidânasthâna* (Pathology). The symptoms and diagnosis of diseases produced by vitiated humours or derangements of blood, bile, wind and phlegm. The symptoms and causes of rheumatic diseases, of piles, stone, fistula-in-ano, leprosy, diabetes, gonorrœah, and ascitcs; the symptoms of unnatural presentative in midwifery, large internal abscess, erysipelas, scrofula, hydrocele, diseases of the organs of generation and of the mouth. These subjects are treated in sixteen chapters.

3rd. *Sarirasthàna* or anatomy. The description of soul and of the elementary parts of the body; of puberty; of conception; of the growth of the different parts of the body; of bleeding; of the treatment of pregnancy and of infants. These subjects are treated in ten chapters.

4th. *Chikitsâsthana*—or Therapia describes the symptoms and treatment of diseases, wounds and ulcers; the history of inflammation; the treatment of fractures, rheumatic diseases, piles, stone, fistula-in-ano, leprosy, diabetes and dropsy; the manner of extracting the child from the uterus in unusual position; the arrangement of diet; remedies for retaining and restoring health and strength, and for prolonging life; the means of preventing diseases; the use of clysters, of errhines and of the smoke of different medicinal substances. All these subjects are treated in forty chapters.

5th. *Kalpasthâna* or the doctrine of antidotes. This explains the means of preparing and preserving food and drink; of distinguishing poisoned food; and descriptions of different mineral, vegetable and animal poisons with their antidotes; they are all treated in eight chapters.

6th. *Uttarasthâna* or the supplementary section. It includes various local diseases not mentioned in the previous chapters, as those of the eyes, nose, ears and head with their treatment; the symptoms and treatment of fever and its varieties; dysentry, consumption, tumours; diseases of the heart, jaundice, discharges of blood and fainting. This is followed by the treatment of intoxication, of cough, hiccough, asthma hoarseness of voice, worms, cholera, dyspepsia and dysuria. It also treats of madness, epilepsy, apoplexy; the different tastes of substances with their effects; the means of retaining health; and the different opinions of praticioners regarding the humours. These are all treated in seventy six chapters.

CHAPTER VIII.

THE RANK OF THE HINDU PHYSICIANS.

In the previous Chapter we have proved that it was the sage Atreya who first instructed pupils in Medical Science. His students were all Brahmins who, as in philosophy, theology and other useful arts and sciences, became equally eminent in medicine. Thus for centuries the Brahmin was the physician, but the manual portion of the profession could not be performed by him pure as he was. To meet this difficulty another caste was formed at a very early period. This was the offshoot of a Brahmin father and a Vaishya mother. The origin of this caste is thus described. The sage Galaba had a maid-servant by name Amba. He was so much pleased with her for her service that he blessed her saying that she should have a son whose name would be *Veerabhadra*,(most fortunate) and that his calling would be that of medicine. This child was called *Ambastha* and his offspring constituted the Vaidya caste who studied the Ayurveda as a profession. This caste was the second in rank and was next to the Brahmins in respect. They studied the Shastras and became learned physicians. Thus the Brahmin studied the Ayurveda for his own enlightenment, the Kshatriya for the benefit of his own health and the Vaidya for his subsistence.

It is seen in a more modern age that some of the Sudras even or the members of the fourth caste learn the Ayurveda when honest and learned.

CHAPTER IX.

THE DUTIES OF THE PHYSICIAN AND HIS ATTENDANTS.

The ancient medical works of the Hindus also give a very beautiful account of how the physicians should behave themselves towards their patients. The Rishis gave a particular stress upon four circumstances relating to the cure of a disease—namely the acquirements of the physician, the proper diagnosis of the disease, proper medicines and good nurses and a reasonable patient. These four circumstances are essentially necessary for the cure of a malady.

First of all a qualified physician is required. The Hindu never placed any confidence in a quack ; learning in a physician was greatly admired. Sushruta thus describes the requirements of a medical practitioner. "He should be of a good family, of healthy body, handsome, pure, vigorous, modest, discrete, patient and intelligent. He should keep his nails and beard short, his body pure and his clothes clean"

It was essentially nessary for a medical man to know well both the theory and practice of his Science. A student knowing the Shastras i e. theoretical portion and not the practical part of the profession is described as " an ass carrying a heavy load of fragrant wood, without discovering and enjoying the fragrance of his burden." If the practitioner does not know his duty well the cure of the desease will be greatly retarded and imperfect.

The nature and temperament of the physician is thus described :—" The physician should always be dignified in his deportment, correct in his manners and habits, gentle and kind, amiable, cheerful and collected. His language should be mild, candid and encouraging, rather like that of a friend than an acquaintance and he should always be ready to assist the sick. His heart should be pure and charitable and he should carefully follow the instructions of his Guru and his predecessors. Such a physician should possess a character for strict veracity, be of calm temper and of the greatest sobriety and chastity. He should be a man of sense and benevolence and his constant thought should he how he is to do good. A person may be afraid of his father and mother, friends and master but not of his physician; so the physician should be more kind and considerate to the sick than a father, a mother, a friend or a master. To these qualities should be added that of affection for learned friends and the constant habit of visiting the sick and seeing them treated by experienced persons.''

These are the qualities which a physician should possess for decoming a successful practitioner. As a professional man he should be acquainted with the causes and varieties of disease and the means of preventing and curing them. A good physician is described as one perfectly acquainted with his own profession. To perform his daily duty he must have a knowledge of (1) *Sutrasthâna* or the relation of customs and habits; (2) *Sarisasthâna*—physiology and anatomy; (3) *Chikitsasthâna* and *Upasaya* or a knowledge of regimen and medicines which cure disease; (4) *Nidânasthâna*—invasion and symptoms of disease; (5) *Upadrava* or unusual symptoms such as delirium, thirst etc.; (6) *Kalpasthâna* or use of poisons.

This list, we dare say, gives an exhaustive account of the amount of theoretical knowledge which a medical practitioner should possess. is not only the theoretical knowledge, to which the Rishis paid every attention, practical knowledge was equally necessary for a medical man. A real and good physician must have in him a combination of theoretical and practical knowledge. Without a knowledge of books a medical man is like a soldier afraid in the time of battle. Such a man, the Shastras enjoin, is a great sinner and should be capitally punished by the Rajah. On the other hand without a practical knowledge a physician's senses will be bewildered when called on to treat acute deseases. Such a person is considered as a murderer—and the medicine, prescribed by him, is like a poison. That a real physician should combine in him both theoretical and practical knowledge is clearly set out by the following simile.

"As the two wheels of a chariot or the two wings of a bird assist in their progress so will the knowledge of the Shastras, and of practice lead the physician to proceed with safety and success in the treatment of the deseased; but should the physician want either of these essential qualities his progress will be impeded as one wing or one wheel will impede the progress of the bird or the chariot."

Thus we see that the ancient Hindus paid equal attention to theoretical and practical knowledge, a combination of which is essential for a good medical practitioner.

The Rishis also laid down beautiful rules of conduct of a physician towards his patient. If a physician is even insultingly and peevishly addressed by a patient he should remain calm, mild and courageous. He should avoid improper and frivolous language particularly with the females. He should not sit down on the same bed with them.

1. How a physician should take up a case and examine his patient is thus described:—the physician should first ask the attendent questions regarding the disease, things the patient has eaten and what he has done to produce or influence the disease. He is then to observe the signs of longivity in the patient. These are long arms and fingers, large eyes, forhead, trunk, teeth, mouth,

hands, feet. Persons will also live to an old age who have long respirations and a large space between the mamillæ, the fore legs short and fleshy and the neck short.

2. The physician should next pay his attention to the nature of the disease, that is he should make a proper and correct diagnosis. In making an accurate diagnosis of the sick person he should observe "his general appearance, the condition of his body, his temperament and strength, the state of the mind and the food he has been used to." He should particularly observe the symptoms of the disease, the state of the pulse, of the tongue as to moisture and dryness, the condition of the bowels, urine and sleep, the general feeling, the state of the nose, head, hands, feet and abdomen, the state of the patient's appetite, the part of the body attacked, the state of the various vessels, the abdomen particularly whether the food is digested. He should also examine the blood, the heart and the lungs.

3. Proper medicines and instruments should be always in hand and the physician

should be well acquainted with them. He should collect drugs from a good soil and neighbourhood. The qualities of the drugs depend on their colour, smell and the kind of juice. The physician should administer good medicines and give directions regarding diet and regimen.

4. He should make selection of good messengers and attandants who contribute a good deal in curing a disease. Such persons should be respectable, courteous, calm, patient and have a knowledge of the Shastras. They should be exact in their description of the cause and progress of the disease and careful that the patient takes the medicine and follows the direction of the physician.

CHAPTER X.

THE PHYSICIAN'S FEES.

As we have written in a previous chapter that the Vaidyas adopted the life of a physician as a means of their live-lihood. The Hindu sages therefore have laid a great stress upon the recompense paid to a physician. They hold that increase of our love to God, our riches, good actions and happiness depends upon the state of our health. Therefore he who cures our desease is a very important person and we should try our very best to pay for his labors. It is thus a religious obligation with every man to pay the fees of his physician. The Shastras enjoin that if a patient does not pay his physician a price equivalent to the value of his soul, then all his holy virtues and good acts which he has performed during his life-time, will belong to the physician. This price, however, is either paid in money or in kind. It is the rich who should make a handsome present of money to his physician which the poor need not do. Money is the recompense paid by the rich, friendship, reputation, increase of virture, prayers and gratitude are that of the poor. How wisely did the ancient Rishis make arrangement for the physician's fees. Every body, rich or poor, stands in need of a medical man's help—he must pay his recompense—the rich may do it with money—the poor with his friendship, prayers or mere gratitude. The physician is also forbidden to accept fees from his spiritual guide, a religious mendicant, a relative, an humble and good friend and one without relations. His duty is to administer medicines for an increase of virtue, fame and happiness as his reward. No better arrangement could have been made by any man for securing medical help for every section of the community.

CHAPTER XI.

HINDU PHYSIOLOGY: GROWTH OF THE HUMAN BODY.

THE human body is the object upon which the Science of Medicine is founded and therefore the Hindu sages paid great attention to its growth. It is thus described by a great oriental scholar :—

"As the mould receives the seed which is to form the future plant, so the menses of the female receive the semen of the male and germination takes place therein. The menses are stated to be of a red colour like the blood of a hare; and they should neither stain cloth when they fall upon it nor have any smell. They are derived from the two vessels of the uterus which discharge their contents, under the influence of the vital air into the uterus and vagina. The menses make their appearance generally about the twelfth year and remain till the fiftieth. At the monthly period the female is moist, plump and happy with her hairs flying about, her eyes languishing, her sides, eyes, arms, breasts, thighs, and navel are in a state of excitement; this period continues for sixteen days when the female may be impregnated. During this time the mouth of the uterus, like the mouth of the rue-fish, is open as the flower of the water-lily when exposed to the sun; as the rays of the light concentrated by a lens produce fire so is generation produced. After this period the mouth of the uterus closes like the petals of the lily when the benign of influence of the sun is absent.

During the period of menses much attention is required regarding the conduct of the woman. During the first three days the woman should remain pure, sit and sleep in purified situation, avoid cold and fatigue and eat temperately. Both parents should be young and healthy. The semen conveyed through the eurethera of the male passes into the vagina, is received into the menses, as a seed, is dropped into a good soil and like it germinates, thus constituting conception. When the mixture has taken place and the resulting body has become solid by the respective qualities of cold and heat the soul is added. When the germ has more the qualities of the semen a male child is formed and when of the menses a female child is the result.

Should conception take place on the first or second day of the menses the child becomes weak and dies soon after birth. If it takes place on the third the child is weak and deformed and dies at an early age. And if it is on the fourth, sixth, eighth or tenth day the child becomes strong and healthy.

The signs of conception described by the Hindu sages are interestingly accurate. During pregnancy the skin round the nipples becomes dark and the hair upon the body becomes more distinct and prominent. The person feels weak, the eyelids are heavy and closed. Much saliva proceeds from the mouth and nose and the woman has no appetite, feels sick and vomits. In this condition a woman must avoid approaching her husband, fasting, vomiting, strong purgatives, grief and fear, scratching and severe coughing, dragging heavy weights, riding on horse back, sleeping during the day and sitting up at night. During pregnancy the woman should be given everything she wants and be kept gratified. How the disposition of the future child is guessed from the desires of the mother is thus described.

"If the woman desires to see a Raja the

child will be great and rich; should the mother wish to adorn herself the child be well-formed and vain; if she wishes to see a holy man the child will be holy and just; if she wishes to see ferocious animals, the child will be of that description."

In the same way the desire of the mother for the various sorts of food gives an idea of the disposition of the child; "if the mother wishes to eat the buffaloe's flesh the child will have blood shot eyes and much hair and will be war-like; and when hog's flesh he will be sluggish and sleepy." The formation of the body and its gradual growth is thus described by the Hindu sages.

"In the first month the mixture of the semen and menses remains like a pea; seven days after conception it has the form of a bubble inflated bag. On the tenth it is red; on the fifteenth it resembles small round piece of flesh. At one month it has small fibres proceeding from it and is animated with life. At the third month the germ becomes of a circular form when a male; of an oblong form when a female; and of an irregular form, when a hermaphrodite. Five eminences begin to appear which when developed become the arms, legs and head. The other smaller parts of the body are then imperfectly formed.

In the fourth month the members are more distinctly developed and the heart being perfectly formed gives the power of sensation and life receives its active powers. In the fifth month the powers of the mind are increased and life performs its usual functions. The nose, mouth, eyes, throat and abdomen may now be distinguished. At the sixth month all the members are formed and the understanding is added. At the seventh month the body is completely formed and the members can act seperately and possess life, mind and understanding. During the eighth month the joints are formed, the parts move on each other, the *foetus* requires food and by the heat of the mother strength is added. At the ninth month the mind and memory are active; it moves about and receives nourishment from the mother. At the tenth month the *foetus* acquires knowledge, prays to God and sees the seven heavens, the earth and the inferior regions.

The signs of immediate delevery are the descent of the uterus and the more flaccid state of the abdomen. The breasts become relaxed and pain commences in the loins, back and inside the thighs with a mucuous discharge.

There are conflicting opinions about which part of the embryo is formed first. Sounaka says that the head is first formed because it is the principal part of all the organs of sense. Kartavirya holds that the heart is first formed because it is the seat of the mind and soul. Parasara says that the Umbilicus is first formed because it is the centre of all other members. Markandeya says that the trunk, the hands and feet are first formed because they are at the root of the active members. Dhanwantari holds that all the members and organs are formed simultaneously.

The internal parts of the foetus are formed in the following manner :—From the elements the eleven senses are produced.

The liver and spleen are formed from the blood; the lungs from its froth; and the intestines from its impurities. Below on the right side is the bladder, the seat of thirst and the root of the urinary vessels; from the blood the gall bladder is replenished with wind. The essential parts of blood and phlegm concocted by the fire of the body into which the wind enters form the intestine, anus and bladder. The tougue is formed from the essential part of blood, phlegm, and flesh. Wind with the assistance of heat seperates the soft parts and forms canals, and passing between the flesh forms the different muscles. When these canals are filled up with marrow they form nerves. The wind entering among the soft parts forms the different receptacles of the body as the stomach and kidneys which are derived from the essential parts of the blood. The testicles and their appendages are formed from the pure part of flesh, blood, phlegm and fat and support of the canals which lead the semen to the pennes. The heart is formed from the essential parts of blood and phlegm and to it all principal arteries are connected.

CHAPTER XII.

THE THREE PERIOD OF A MAN'S LIFE.

The Hindu Physician has divided a man's life into three periods, namely childhood, manhood and decrepitude. The first extends up to the fifteenth year when phlegm is in excess. Manhood extends from the sixteenth to the seventieth year while bile is in excess. This age is again divided into a period of growth which extends from the sixteenth to the twentieth year; of youth from the twentieth to the thirtieth year; of maturity from the thirtieth to the fortieth year when all the humours, senses, strength are in full development; and of weakness from the fortieth to the seventieth year when all the powers of the organs are gradually diminishing and bile is in excess. Decrepitude extends from the seventieth year till the person's death; during this period the humours, senses, strength and animation daily diminish. In this period of life air is in excess and nervous diseases prevail.

After the tenth year memory, feeling, sight, semen, strength and the active senses are powerful; the growth of the body after twenty years and the perfect state of the body after thirty years. The males are supposed to arrive at their perfection in figure and strength at twenty-five and the females at sixteen years of age.

CHAPTER XIII.

STRUCTURE OF THE BODY.

According to the Hindu Medical Science the human body is made up of six members consisting of four extremeties, the trunk and the head. The regions are ether single or double; the former are the head, front, back, umbilicus, chest, abdomen, chin and neck; the double are the ears, eyes, nostrils, supercilia, temples, cheeks, shoulders, mammæ, testes, sides, nates, knees, arms, legs &c. There are also ten fingers, ten toes and the organs of sense. The body has nine orifices like a house with doors. They are the uretha, anus, mouth, nostrils, eyes, and ears; the vagina forms the tenth in the female. This is the general division of the body. The particular parts of the body are seven membranes, seven regions, seven elementary bodies, humours and secretions; also the liver, spleen, lungs, kidneys, heart, anus, intestines, præcordia, organ of sense, large vessels, urinary, gall bladder, hair ligaments, sutures, commissures of bones, capsular membranes, bones, joints, tendons, muscles, vital parts, vessels, nerves and organs producing unions.

The above is the general structure of the body described by the Hindu sages. They have also given particular descriptions of the different parts proving conclusively their knowledge of anatomy and physiology. We will first give a particular account of the various humours of the body. The food that is taken into the stomach has portions of elements in it; when they are mixed by digestion they constitute the humours of the human body. These are considered the pillars of the body and consist of *Vayu* (wind) *Pitta* (bile) and *Kaph* (phlegm). The *Vayu* or wind flows through all parts of the body and performs all its actions. It carries the essential parts about the body, performs respiration, all the actions at the outlets of the body. There are, according to the Hindu sages, five kinds of wind in a human body: (1) *Prâna*, vital: it passes through the mouth and nose and performs deglutition. It lies in the chest and is the supporter of life. works the blood, conveys food and drink to the stomach and strength to the body. When deseased it produces hiccough, difficulty of breathing etc. (2) *Apâna*: it lies in the rectum, uretha, buttock &c., and is situated in the place of digestion. It separates urine, semen, menses and expels the fœtus. When diseased it produces diseases of the bladder and anus, semen and constipation. (3) *Shamana*: it lies in the stomach and small intestines. It digests the blood and separates blood and juices from the urine, alvine evacuations &c. When diseased it produces loss of appetite, goolmoh, diarrhæa &c. (4) *Udana*: it exists in the hollow of the neck, above the sternum and always goes upwards. It produces speech, singing and other functions of the voice above the collar bones. When deranged it produces various diseases of the upper part of the chest and neck. (5) *Vyâna*: it conveys fluids over the body. It causes the flow of blood, sweat &c., and performs ; walking, jumping, opening of the eyes &c. If diseased all the body becomes affected.

Pitta (bile) is a hot, bitter, oily fluid having a peculiar smell like that of raw flesh. It is of a blue colour when in a state of digestion, is sour, pungent, bitter and light in weight when unmixed; and of a yellow colour when properly prepared. It produces animal heat. It lies in the stomach and small intestines—and is also found in the liver, spleen, heart, eye and skin where it is mixed with blood and other fluids. There are five kinds of bile:—(1) *Pacheka*: it is situated between the stomach and small intestines; it is bodily fire produced by the five elements. It digests the food and separates, the chyle, urine and fæces. (2) *Ranjaka*: it is situated in the liver and spleen; it gives the blood-red colour to chyle. (3) *Shadaka*: it exists in the heart and produces sense, memory and thought. (4) *Atochoka*: it exists in the eye and produces sight. (5) *Brajoka*: it exists in the skin and gives it a shining and healthy colour.

When not deranged bile produces the sense of sight, digestion and the function of organs, by its heating and concocting properties. It produces appetite and thirst and retains the body soft giving the proper colour to it; and also produces joy, pride memory etc. When it is deranged the internal fire or heat of the body is diminished as also its colour and digestion. In this case, the nourishing chyle (rasa) is not properly separated in the organ called amassia and produces the undigested dejections called ama or white slimy discharges.

The phlegm (*Kaph*) is the impurity of the chyle and is conveyed by the *prâna vayu* along the *domonnie* vessels and mixes with the rest of the phlegm in the body. It is cooling, moist, white, heavy, oleaginous and glistening. It is sweet, but when imperfectly digested becomes pungent, prepared by the internal fire as if boiled in an earthen pot. If deranged by fire it becomes saltish and frothy. It is principally found in the stomach, in the breast, in the heart, at the root of the neck, in the head, in the eyes, in the throat and the tongue. There are five kinds of this (*Kapha*) (phlegm) described :—

1. In the stomach *(amassia)* phlegm softens the food, retains chyle of its proper consistence and pervades and strengthens the different organs.

2. *Avalamvana* is situated in the heart, shoulder, joint and arms and strenghens these parts and the breast.

3. In the tongue and throat it produces

the various tastes, such as bitter, salt, and sour and is called *rashana.*

4. In head it keeps, by its lubricating qualities, the brain, the eyes and other organs moist. It is called *Strehena.*

5. It keeps the joints moist and ready, to perform their actions and is called *Shlesona.*

We will now describe what the Hindu physicians speak of the essential parts or *Dhâtu.* They are the supporters of the body and consist of the hard and soft parts and fluids of the body. These are chyle *(rasa)*, blood (*rakta*), flesh (*mânsa*), fat (*meda*), bone (*asthi*) marrow (*majjâ*) and semen (*Sukra*). These seven essential parts of the body form the fœtus, lubricate the food, nourish and sustain life and retain the system in a healthy state; they give the soft feel, colour and strength to the body and the action of the senses. When deseased or diminished the body wastes and the person dies. Charaka and Sushruta disagree about the number of bones. The former say they are 306 and the latter 300. This shows how carefully the Hindus examined the human body.

They next speak of *Malá* or excretions. These are the dregs or impurities of the seven essential parts. The dregs of the chyle is phlegm; that of the blood, bile; of the flesh, the secretions of the ear, nose etc; of the fat perspirartion; of the bone, the nails and hair; of the brain and marrow, the secretions from the eyes etc; the semen has no dregs, but others say that ozah, an oily transparent fluid, which is spread over the body, and is its essential support, is its impurity.

As regards joints or *Sandhi* the Hindu Physicians differ. According to Susruta there are 107 articulations; others state there are 68 joints moveable, and 142 immoveable, of the moveable kind are the joints of the extremeties, jaw, and vertebrae. All the others belong to the second or immoveable class.

The Hindu Physicians next speak of *Snaya* or ligaments. Ligaments bind together and strengthen the flesh, fat, joints and frame work of the body, like the strips of ratan which are employed to bind the pieces of a boat together. Susruta enumerates 900 ligaments; divided into 600 of the extremeties, 230 of the trunk and 70 of the neck and head. There are four varieties of ligaments :—

1. *Pratanobutee*, long ligaments and tendons, as of the legs, feet and joints.

2. *Britto*, round ligaments and tendons, as of the penis etc.

3. *Prithu*, thick ligaments and tendons as along the sides, breast, back and head.

4. *Susira* are hollows, as in *amassia*, *pukassia* and bladder.

Next comes muscles or *Pashee*. They cover, strengthen and retain the vessels, tendons, bones and joints in their places. Susruta describes them as five hundred. Then come the vessels. From the navel proceed all the vessels and it is the principal seat of life. Susruta enumerates forty principal vessels and distinguishes 700 branches. These are divided into three classes, which differ more in their offices, than in their appearance. They are *Shira*, *Dhamanee* and *Srota*.

The *Shira* vessels are numerous and of all sizes and convey wind, bile, phlegm, and blood to all parts of the body. They convey nourishment throughout the body as a garden is irrigated by a small brook. *Dhamanee* vessels include the large vessels and nerves which proceed from the navel by which the functions of hearing, touch, sight, taste and smell are performed. There are twenty-four of these vessels, according to Sushruta which proceed from the navels. *Srota* are canals. There are many canals in the human frame which assist the nervous and vital powers. These convey *Prana* or vital air, food, water chyle, blood, fat of the flesh, urine, faces, semen and menses.

Next come the *Jálas* the circular tissue that connects and surrounds the different parts of the body and retains the seven essential parts such as the blood, bile, etc., separate from each other. There are, according to the Hindu physicians, seven kinds of *Jàlas*.

Then follow the *Asaya* or receptacles. These are seven with an additional three in the female. They retain the humours of the body in their respective situations. The receptacle of the blood is the heart under which is stomach. Under this is *Pakâsaya* receptacle of bile, below which is the *Pavanashaya* the receptacle of urine. The female has three receptacles, the uterus and the two mammæ.

In this way the Hindu physicians have given accurate description of the skin and the vital parts or *marma.*

From the above accounts it is clear that the ancient Hindu physicians were well read in physiology and practical anatomy. For this purpose all the Rishis are said to have recommended the dissection of the human body as proper and necessary. Charaka says that a practitioner should know all the parts of the body both external and internal and their relative positions with regard to each other. Even the great legistator Manu has laid down that one touching a corpse is purified by a bathing. Sushruta says that a holy man should dissect in order that he may know the different parts of the body and a surgeon and physician should not only know the external appearances, but the internal structure of the body too. Thus we see that the ancient Hindu physicians were also well read in anatomy and their proficiency in practical anatomy was perfected by the dissection of the human body. In the ancient medical works, etc., we also find rules laid down for dissection and they have always recommended the dead body of a healthy person for the purpose.

CHAPTER XIV.

HINDU MATERIA MEDICA.

The early Hindu physicians believed that there is a remedy for each disease. This led the Hindu sages to make a very careful examination of the vegetable, animal and mineral kindoms. And by this means they discovered a number of medicines some of which were very powerful.

The simple vegetable medicines are procured from the bark, roots, leaves, flowers, fruits, seeds, juices, gums and wood of plants. The effects of medicines from the vegetable kingdom vary with the period at which they are gathered according as this takes place in windy or calm-whether, in sunshine or in the shade, during the day or night, in cold or hot whether, in a dry or rainy season. They have also given a description of the place from which medicines should be gathered ; they should be procured from a fruitful country where the soil is soft and moist, of a black, yellow and red colour, of an equable weight, situated near water where trees grow luxuriantly.

Medicines prepared from the animal kingdom are also equally valuable.

1. Skin ; nails and hair are used for fumigations in intermittent fevers.

2. Blood ; when there has been a great loss of blood it is sometimes exhibited internally.

3. Flesh is mixed with oily and other medicines and vegetables , and is given in weakness, pthysis and nervous diseases.

4. Bones, the ashes of bones, mixed with other medicines are exhibited in nervous diseases and those of children. They are also used to fumigate.

5. Oils and fats are used principally externally as in the form of ointment &c.

6. Marrow is used externally in the form of ointment and internally in cases of weakness.

7. Bile is considered a stimulant and is used in fever; also as an external application to the eyes.

8. Milk is one of the principal articles of food.

9. Urine is slightly laxative and cures diseases of phlegm and wind and diseases produced by worms or from poison. It is also of use in leprosy and in dropsical swellings, jaundice and dyspepsia.

10. Dung. The moisture used in cow's dung is used in inflammation and in discolourations of the skin.

The Hindu physicians were the first who employed mineral drugs internally. They knew how to prepare sulphuric, nitric and muriatic acids. This shows that the science of Chemistry was known to the Hindus earlier than to any other nation even the Arabs. Mineral medicines consist of salts, precious stones, poisons and metals.

Thrse are four kinds of salts used in medicine: saltpetre, natron, black salt and borax. Common salt is stomachic and cures wind and indigestion. Natron or impure carbonate of soda is advantageously employed in dyspepsia, cholic and enlargement of the spleen. They cure swellings, piles, dysentry and stone.

Certain precious stones and earthly minerals are supposed to possess superior qualities as tonics and corroborants. The diamond is the chief of these of which they distinguish four varieties—the white, yellow, red and black. Pearls, corals and other precious stones are prepared by mixing them with lemon juice for a day, boiling them in the juice of the three varieties of myrobalans and exposing them to heat covered with a coating of clay and cow dung when they are ready for use. They are considered great tonics and cure many diseases.

The metals which were employed by the ancient Hindu physicians were mercury, gold silver, copper, lead, tin, zinc, antimony, carbonate of iron and arsenic. The preparations of quick-silver with zinc, antimony, and arsenic were probably introduced into Hindustan at a very early period. The purification of quick-silver was prescribed in the following way :—

To purify quick-silver from lead mix it in rice-water and expose it to fire. To purify it from tin mix it with powder of Vishāl (cucumis colocynthis) and ankotha (alangium henapetalum) and expose it to fire. To purify it from other impurities, add the juice of cassia fistula and when in globules mix it with the juice of Datura and lime and then expose it to heat.

Similarly to purify mercury, take of turmeric, brick-dust, suet, the juice of lemons and the wool of sheep, of each one chatak and mix it with one *sheer* of quick-silver. The mixture is to be well rubbed in a mortar for one day and the product carefully washed with water and acidulated with fermented rice water.

Gold, like other metals intended for medicinal purposes, was first reduced by hammering to small thin plates. These were exposed to a red heat, and in this state cooled first in oil, then in curdled milk, cow's urine, tea-water and decoction of *Kulattka*.

The perparations of gold are considered as most valuable medicines, curing nearly all diseases. The general effect, of these preparations, is to increase memory and restore the vigour of manhood, improve the natural colour of the body, retain the proper equilibrium of the different internal parts of the body; and so lengthen vision and prolong life.

The usual manner of preparing gold for use is to mix sixteen times the quantity of the gold plates to one of lead and add lemon juice or *ghritacumari* or Indian aloes. They are to be rubbed together, exposed to heat and made into boluses, of the usual size; or take the mass of gold plates, mix with quick-silver and sulphur, add a little water or the juice of *ghritacumari*, make it into a large mass; put it in an earthen pot, with its mouth well-secured, surround the vessel with a mixture of clay and cow-dung and expose it to the sun to dry. It is thus to be exposed to the fire twelve different times until it is reduced to powder.

Silver is prepared by mixing two parts of it reduced to small thin plates with one of brimstone and one of the sulphuret of arsenic. It is to be prepared in the same way as gold. It lengethens life and is of much use in all chronic diseases.

Copper is purified by boiling it for three days with a strong heat the small thin plates in cow's urine. The metal is then to be mixed with two parts of brimstone and one part of rock salt to which the juice of lemon is to be added. The mixture, then surrounded with a coating of clay and cow-dung, is to be exposed to the fire of furnace.

The sulphate of copper is prepared by mixing two parts of the thin plates with one of sulphar. It is then to be exposed to heat with free exposure to the air for two hours. These preparations are useful in fevers, diarrhœa, diseases of the liver, spleen and blood, leprosy, colic, piles, acidity, dyspepsia and rheumatism.

Lead is used in the form of the carbonate, the red oxide and litharge and prepared for use by mixing it with the juice of the *Akanda* tree. It should remain immersed for three days; then wash the metal in water, mix it with the juice of the leaves of the Vasaka tree and sulphur. Put it in an earthen pot and expose it to a high degree of diet. It is used in Gonorrhœa, in chronic diarrhœa, in worms, leprosy and ulcers.

Similarly they have given accounts of numerous other metalic preparations which now appear wonderful to the modern chemists.

CHAPTER XV.

THE HINDU PHARMACY.

1. *Weights and measures*—The Hindu physicians used the following weights. One

Soorkh equal to 1 grain; one *masha*=8 *Soorkhas* (or gr. VIII); one direm, equal to 3 *mashas* (grs XXIV); 1 tola equal to 12½ mashas; 2 tolas=a karsha or aksha. It should be noted here that a tola in the ancient sanskrit Mss. is equal to a half a tola of the modern medical weights.

The fluid measure consists of a pot made of bamboo, wood or iron called *Kudeva*; a measure of capacity, the sixth part of a maund and the fourth of a *prastha* or a vessel four inches in diameter and as many deep.

The modern Bengali physicians consider the tola or one sicca Rupee weights. It weighs 180 English troy, weight grains. 8 tolas=1 pala; 2 palas=1 prassitis or hand-ful; 5 tolas=1 chatack; 4 chattaks=powah; 4 powahs=1 seer and 40 Seers=1 mds.

2. *Preparation of medicines.*—The Hindus used iron or stone mortars which were used cold, or heated by exposure to a fire made of the dry utter of goats or husks of rice. The pestle was either of iron or

earthenware; of sufficient size to hold by the hand.

3. *Form of medicines:*—Internal medicines are usually used in the form of powders the juice of plants, pastes, infusions, decoctions, extracts, roasted medicines, tincturis, pills, electuaries, medicines that are sucked and oils.

In making powders dry them in the sun or over fire, powder them in a mortar and then clean it by passing it through a sieve. The fresh juice of plants is also frequently used, is got from the leaves and is prepared by boiling it. Pastes are prepared by grinding the medicine between two stones. *Infusions* are prepared by mixing one part of green or soft medicines with four parts of boiling water. For preparing decoctions take two *tolas* of the medicine to half a seer of water, or one part to sixteen parts of water and boil down to one quarter. For making extracts make a decoction of the medicine in water, boil for a certain time, strain it through linen and again boil it down until it becomes thick. Too much boiling should be avoided and the test is that when a small portion is thrown into water it does not mix in it. *Electuaries* are preparations made by boiling down the decoction of medicine to one quarter and mixing sugar with it, again boiling for some minutes and when it has arrived at the consistence of congealing quickly on being removed from the fire adding the prescribed powders.

4. The Hindu physicians also paid much attention to the administration of medicines: they laid down the following precepts regarding it.

(1). In short and accute diseases the medicine is to be taken in an empty stomach that it may be sooner digested. (2) The medicine may be taken with advantage before eating when the patient is strong and disease severe. (3) One-half of the medicine should be taken before and another after food. (4) By the old and weak the medicine should be taken with the food. (5) By others after the food when the disease has occurred suddenly and when the patient suffers from asthma, cough, thirst and vomitting. (6)

Another kind should be taken with a covering over it. (7) When the disease is in the middle of the body, the medicine is to be taken between the two periods of eating. (8) Another kind of medicine should taken with each morsel of food. (9) For asthma, cough, thirst, etc., an emetic should be occasionally administered.

5. *Classification and uses of drugs.*—Charaka arranges drugs under forty-five heads, according to their action in removing classes of symptoms. Sushruta divides medicines into two classes, one of which increases strength, by evacuating bad humours from the body as purgatives and emetics; and the other lowers the exalted action of the humours and restores them to a healthy state. By another arrangement medicines are classified accordingly as they are supposed to cure wind, bile and phlegm, according to their action on certain organs, for the treatment of certain diseases or classes of symptoms.

Thirty-nine simple drugs are enumerated for curing diseased wind, twenty-three for curing diseased phlegm, and twenty for deranged bile.

Medicines may be usefully arranged, according to their actions into diaphoratics, emetics, purgatives, pastes, enemata, errhines, diuretics, astringents, tonics, emollients, nutrients, maturants, &c. The Hindu physician, before any of these medicines were given, relaxed the body, by rubbing oil upon it externally and giving some oleaginous mixture internally.

1. Diaphoretics were the application of heat; by the steam of hot water; by the application of certain warm poultices, or plasters, made of different medicines: and by fomentations, with various decoctions. For promoting perspiration, the body should be relaxed by the use of ghee, oil, fat, and marrow. Of these, ghee is the best, as it is produced from milk obtained from the cow. This milk first yields curdled milk, then butter, and with the assistance of fire, ghee is produced. Nothing else can be obtained from ghee, so that it may be considered as pure. For diseases of the bile, ghee only is

to be given; of wind, ghee and salt, mixed; and for, diseases of phlegm, ghee, long-pepper, pepper, dry ginger, and nitre, mixed together. A weak person, with a bad memory and digestion, should use ghee to strengthen them. In certain cutaneous diseases, for open boils and for worms, oil is useful, particularly when the phlegm is deranged. To fat people, particularly when the wind is deranged, and when the dejections are not natural oil should be first given. Lard is most useful for external diseases, those of the joints, bones, and sensible parts.

Perspiration should not be promoted in the scrotum, throat, or eyes. When wind and phlegms are deranged, diaphoretic medicines that contain the qualities of coldness and heat respectively are to be used. When wind is deranged, cooling medicines alone are to be used. When wind and phlegm are deranged in a part, or when only wind or phlegm is deranged, perspiration is to be promoted in such places alone.

Perspiration is not to be encouraged in very fat, very thin, or debilitated persons, when affected with diseases of the blood or wind; when the diseases are incurable; in dysentery; or when the person is afflicted with large sores over the body (Kotha). Nor will perspiration be proper after taking poisons, or drinking, or for the blind; when the abdomen is swelled; or in erysipelas, or leprosy, or in a bad state of the blood. In such cases milk, ghee, curdled milk, and honey should be given after purgatives.

It is improper to give diaphoretics when the body is burnt; in diseases of anus; in grief, or fear-producing diseases; in passions, in hunger, in thirst, in weakness, in jaundice, in gonorrhœa, in hemoptysis, in pulmonary consumption, in dysentery, during the flow of the menses, or after taking much wine; in pregnancy, particularly near its termination; in diseases of wind, or in fatal diseases. When diaphoretics are used under such circumstances, they will do harm, or their peculiar favourable effects will not be produced.

After oleaginous and perspiring medicines have been exhibited, any of the other five varieties of medicines may be employed with advantage, according to the effect that is required to be produced.

2. Emetics and purgatives are supposed to be the most powerful medicines when the wind, bile, and phlegm are moderately diminished or deranged, and they restore the humours to their healthy state. In general, emetics are recommended when the stomach is surcharged with phlegm; and purgatives, when the intestines and bile are deranged.

When the practitioner has decided on the necessity of giving an emetic, the preliminary relaxing medicines, with honey and saindhabha (an impure kind of salt), are to be exhibited. This is usually done in the morning, or the day before the exhibition of the emetic; more particularly when the strength and internal heat of the person are great, and the humours much deranged. The patient should then drink freely of milk, whey, rice, or water, or the like. The emetic should be given, and the warm hand applied frequently to the abdomen, for an hour, to soften it. If it cannot be taken in the usual way, by means of its taste, it may be sucked through the stalk of a hollow reed, so that it may pass down the throat. The emetic should be taken in the morning. The person is to place himself upon a stool, with his thigh parallel to the floor, and his head, back, and sides supported by friends. He will first feel sick, then saliva will follow from his mouth, and tears, and mucus from his eyes, and nose, followed by vomiting. The vomiting will be promoted by thrusting the finger, or the stalk of a lily, down the throat. The vomiting is to be encourged until the stomach is completely emptied; this is known to be the case, by the discharge of the saliva, by the bad breath, and by the body being itchy.

Among the emetics, madana fruit (spermacoce hispida) is the best, and may be administered in the form of powder or decoction, with honey and rocksalt. An emetic is sometimes prepared bruising and mixing long peper, Indian sesamum (teta), indrogobo, saindhava (impure salt), and the root of the moina tree (madana). The vangueria spinosa, asclepias, germinata, azadirachta (the Indian species of mustard); bitter cucurbitacea, fossil-salt, and the sulphate of copper, mixed with several vegetable drugs, were employed mixed with honey, as an emetic, which was recommended to be used when poison has been taken.

3. Purgatives. The day before a common purgative is exhibited, the patient is required to eat light food in combination with warm water, so as to remove any derangement of the phlegm. The next morning the body is anointed with oil, and exposed to heat, to promote perspiration, after which, the purgative is administered, and is supposed to clear the body of diseased humours below the stomach. It is stated that should this preparation not be attended to, the person's constitution will be injured. These purgatives should be varied according to the state of the bowels, and the purpose for which they are given.

First, when there is looseness with much bile, the medicine should be cool and in small quantities.

Secondly, when wind and phlegm are deranged with costiveness, the medicine acts with difficulty, and should be exhibited warm and strong.

Thirdly, there is a middle condition in which the bile, wind, and phlegm are affected with the bowels, neither constipated, nor relaxed, in which case the medicine should be given of a temperate heat, and of moderate quantity and quality.

The dose of aperient medicine should vary with the age, &c., of the patient, and when a purgative has been administered, in the above form, its action should not be suddenly stopped. The patient should stay in a closed room, and he should not take cold water, nor use force in the evacuation. When the purgative has not produced the desired effect, it will cause derangement in the bile and phlegm. The body is hot, there is no appetite—and there is a heaviness in the belly, uneasiness in the breast, itchiness of the arms and not a free evacuation of the urine.

Purgatives should not be given during the beginning of the fever; that is, while the patient feels a slight appetite and his bowels are not very costive. For infants, and old or very fat people, purgatives are to be avoided; also when the body is very hot or much fatigued; in bloody stools, and immediately after labour; also when the appetite is bad, in derangement of the blood, bile and wind, when there are sores on the body, or internally, when there is great thirst, after loss of blood; and in diseases of the lungs. Should a quack give purgatives at an improper time he will kill the person.

Purgatives should be used in fevers, in diseases from poisons, in piles, in swelling of the glands, in jaundice, in epilepsy, in diseases of the heart, in fiistula-in-ano, in vomiting, in diseases of the vagina, in colicky pains, in costiveness, and in cholera; in certain disease of the belly (alasaka), in leprosy, in eruptions, in gonorrhœa, in the enlargement of the spleen, in hydrocele, in ophthalmia, and in general diseases of the eye, especially in purulent ophlhalmia; in diseases of the head, ear and nose, in those of the anis and penis, in worms, in diseases of the bile, involuntary discharges of semen, and &c.

The discharge produced by purgatives are first, urine, fæces, bile, then the medicine, and lastly phlegm.

Of the purgatives the trivrit, or as is it usually called teori (convolvulus turpethum) and Haritaki (chebulic myrobalan) are considered the best. Of the oily purgatives, the castor oil is the best. In diseases of wind, give teori in powder (6 annas weight for a dose) with the juice of the sugar cane, danti (croton polyandrum), ricinus communis, cassia fistula, purgative cucurbitaceœ, the seed of ipomœa cœrulea, myrobolans, the juice of euphorbia antiqusrum; along with these sugar, fruits, &c, are used as laxatives and combined with warm aromatics, such as pepper, ginger, &c.

In diseases of the bile, the medicine is administered with milk; and in diseases of phlegm, the same medicine is given with the decoction of long and black pepper and dry ginger.

The covering of the Haritaki, is to be

used like the teori, in the same form and dose, and to cure the same diseases. Castor oil is prepared by gathering the seed at the proper season, drying it for seven days, and taking the kernels and boiling them in water the oil is to be removed for use—in other cases the oil is got by pressing the seeds between weights. This oil is to be given the children from birth to the tenth year. It is also given to old and weak and delicate persons.

Purgatives may be prepared and exhibited with ghee, oil, milk, wine, cow's urine, broths, and certain form of food. The action of purgative medicines will be increased by using warm water with some infusion, the warm or vapour bath, and friction with the warm hand. When the laxative effect is not sufficient, it is not to be repeated till the next day; but when a sufficient effect has been produced the purgatives should not be repeated for ten days.

A small dose of purgative should be first given, and when the individual's constitution is better known, a stronger one may be administered. The following are examples of purgative mixtures: take of Haritaki (yellow myrobalon), salt, and long pepper, in equal proportions; grind them into a paste with water; dose three drams. Or, take of Haritaki (yellow myrobalan), and amalaki, (emblic myrobalan), vibhitaki (beleric myrobalan) in equal parts: three tolas of this mixture are to be boiled in forty-eight of water, until reduced to twelve tolas. To six tolas of this infusion add three of castor oil. Or take three tolas (nine drams) of castor oil, with six of milk. The purgative is varied according as the wind, phlegm, and bile, are deranged.

Another class of medicines, produce both vomiting and purging; they are—kashataki, several sorts of cucurbitaceous plants, saptala, (abrus precatorius); shankhini (cissampelos hexandra); devadani rubitaki (fruit and bark), ravilika (momordica charantika). The juices of these plants are used for producing their effects, as the organs of speech for the articulation of vowels and sibilants.

4. Pastes composed of different purga-

tive drugs were often used with great benefit. The following is an example, and was applied to the navel: Take of ras, quicksilver; gomdak, sulphur; marick, black pepper, of each a quarter tola; sohaga, biborate of soda; pippoli, long pepper; shanthi, dry ginger, of each half a tola; dantibit, croton polyandrum, two and a quarter tolas; mix into a paste with the milky juice of seejor (enphorbium longifolium). Put in into the milk of a cocoa-nut, which is to be coated with clay, and expose it to fire for two hours until the clay is red hot, and when cooled the dose of the paste is two tolas.

5. Enemeta. This is considered as the best manner of exhibiting purgative medicines in diseases of the lower part of the abdomen, and lower extremities. Medicines may thus be mixed so as to cure diseases of wind, bile, and phlegm, as the medicine enters the system like water poured at the root of a tree. These medicines were much used by the ancient practitioners.

The general effect of enemas is to strengthen the muscles, and to lessen fat. They retain the eyes and surface in a healthy state —and will retain the body healthy till death, or even lengthen the period of existence.

The bladders of pigs, buffalos, &c., are used for these injections. For this purpose the animal should be healthy, and of full age. Should bladders not be found a leather bag may be substituted. The injecting pipe should be made of gold, silver, copper, iron, hard wood, or ivory. It should be smooth, strong, and tapering like the tail of a cow, with a slightly tuberculated extremity, six finger's breadth in length to the cross piece, for patients from the first to the eighth year of age; eight or ten from the ninth to the sixteenth year; and afterwards somewhat longer. During the first years, the tube should the size of the little finger, afterwards of the ring finger, then of the middle finger; and after the twenty-fifth year, the size of the thumb, in administering enemata, care must be taken not to introduce it in an oblique direction, nor too far nor too short a distance, and not to press it on one side. The size of the injection should also be varied, according to the size of the patient's hands.

For the very young, two handsful of the liquid are to be used, for a child of eight years, four, and from sixteen upwards, eight hands-ful.

There are two varieties of glysters, one without and another with oil. The first form of enemata should be prepared with honey and ghee ; animal and vegetable broths should likewise be administered. The following is offered as an example of a glyster in costiveness, piles, dyspepsia, intermittent fever, in diseases of the loins, back, and intestines. It should be prepared as following :—

Take of the decoction of suttee ; pushkara, a kind of costus ; krishnapaka, cariss carondas ; madan, datura, metal ; dubdaru, uvaria longifolia, kushtha, costus speciousus ; yasti madhu, liquorice ; villa, assafœtida ; and ten parts of milk and four of oil ; mix and administer warm. Various other glysters are prepared in much the same way.

This form of administering medicine is is very useful when not too frequently employed in fever, diarrhœa, and dysentery; in diseases of the head, and eyes; in tetanus; in convulsions, and in many nervous and other diseases.

Enemata are not proper for the very young, or very old, for the timid, or those labouring under grief, for women before the third or fourth month of pregnancy, in madness, in piles, jaundice, in fainting, in indigestion, in vomiting, leprosy, dropsy, asthma, cough, diseases of the throat, diseases of wind, such as swelling of the extremities, or in nervous diseases.

Injections by the urethra. These should be used by a tube fourteen fingers' breadth in length, with an opening of the size to allow a mustard seed to pass. For the females, the tube should be four finger's breadth in length, and the opening capable of allowing the passage of small pea. The tube should be covered with oil, and gently introduced, while pressure is made on the bladder, over the pubis, and the marks fixed on the tube prevents its being introduced too far. The injection should be two tolas in quantity;

and is used for diseases of the semen, of the bladder, and the uterus.

When there is a burning in the bladder, an injection of honey, sugar, or a decoction of liquoria and cold water is given. In some cases injections of ghee are used, and in others, astringent injections, such as decoctions of the bark of the banian tree. After the introduction of the injection, the patient should take bland drinks, such as barley, water, congee, or animal broths.

The evacuation by purgatives, emetics, enemata, and blood-letting, leaves the patient with the internal fire diminished, and on that account heavy food should be avoided, and light and nourishing food taken.

6. Errhines. This is a large class of local irritants, and they are used with the intention of producing sneezing, and exciting a discharge from the nostrils by which the head is supposed to be cleared from the presence of bad humours.

There are four varieties of fumes used as errhines:—

1. The varieties of smoke are taken by

the nostrils at three efforts. For this purpose different spices are ground into powder, and a tube is used twelve fingers' breadth in length, the size of the little finger at one end, and tapering to the size of the thumb at the other, with an aperture of the size of the small pea. For eight fingers' breadth the tube on the inside, is to be covered with silk cloth, over which the medicine is rubbed. The tube, thus prepared, is to be set fire to, and the fumes are to be drawn into the nostrils.

2. Only masses, made with wax, different gums, such as gum-resin, with ghee, are lighted, and the fumes are received into the nostril.

3. Those which clear the head, are made with medicines which irritate the nostrils, such as black pepper, long pepper, and aguru, a kind of fragrant wood. These are to be made into a paste, with which the tube is covered, and then lighted. The fumes produce the effect desired.

4. Those which cause vomiting, are formed by burning the skin and hair of animals, dry fish and flesh, and substances

which produce vomiting. The smoke should be taken in first by the mouth and evacuated through the nostrils, and when taken by the nostrils it should be passed through the mouth.

These are the usual forms in which errhines are given for promoting the secretion of the mucous membrane of the glottis, trachea, and air cells of the lungs. In diseases of the throat and chest, the smoke is to be taken by the mouth; and by the nose, when the head, nose, and eyes are affected. Some are employed to cure cough.

These medicaments are prepared with sugar, the juice of the sugar-cane, milk, ghee, and animal broths, which clear the head. They are used for diseases of the heart, as in fainting; and for weak and delicate persons. Those prepared with medicines which clear the head of pent-up humours, accompanied with weight and pain of the head, are usually of an oily nature; and are introduced into the nostrils by means of a tube. This form is likewise used in diseases of the throat, particularly swelling, when warms infest the head and nose; in jaundice; in polypus of the nose, when the person can neither distinguish taste nor smell, oily substances are usually employed. It is used in diseases of the mouth, eye, and ear, caused by derangements of the phlegm.

Errhines, prepared to clear the head, are used in the form of powder, and in health, after waking from sleep, after fatigue, both in the morning and evening. These medicines are used in epilepsy, apoplexy, and other diseases producing a loss of sense, and cure diseases above the neck, and retard the marks of old age.

When phlegm is deranged, the errhines are to be given in the morning; when bile; at noon; and when the wind is deranged, in the evening.

Errhines should not be employed in hœmoptysis, after emetics and purgatives, in swelling of the abdomen (Udara) in involuntary discharges of the semen, in sudden blindness, and when the wind is deranged after eating much food, or drinking wine; after poisons, wounds, or injuries of the head; in jaundice, when the person cannot sleep, or when he is very thirsty.

Fumigations. Sores are frequently recommended to be fumigated. For this purpose a tube is used eight fingers' breadth in length, and the fumes of the medicines are to be conveyed so as to be brought into contact with the surface of the sores.

7. Gargles. The quantity should be such as can be moved about in the mouth. The patient should stand erect. He should attend to what he is doing, and when the fluid is mixed with the bad humours of the mouth, nose, or eyes, it is to be evacuated, and another portion is to be taken in the mouth. Gargles usually consist of astringent decoctions, or the juice of acid fruits, black pepper, long pepper, dry ginger, vacha, mustard, mixed with oil, vinegar, wine, cow's urine, salt or honey, according to disease, &c. They may be used either hot or cold, and when properly employed, they cure diseases of the mouth, clean it, and sooth the part.

8. Emmenagogues. The remedies for restoring or bringing on the menstrual dis-

charge, are vinegar and acids, cow's urine, curdled milk, and wine. They are not often used, and as the irregularies are often produced by weakness, tonics are frequently given.

9. Diuretics. This important class of medicines is used in stranguary, in pain of the bladder, in scanty urine, and in gravel and stone. They are used either in decoction or in powder.

10. Parturifacients. Medicines for promoting the expulsion of the fœtus from the womb, were not known by the Hindu practitioners. In cases of lingering labour, manipulation used to be employed to advance delivery.

11. Sialogogues. Medicines for increasing the secretion from the mouth when too dry, were often had recourse, to for expelling morbid humours from its neighbour-hood. They should never be used before the fifth year of age. The chief medicines belonging to this class, are calomel and corrosive sublimate. The other medicines of this class, are black and long pepper, dry ginger,

rock salt, acid fruits, vaçha, and other hot spices.

12. Stimulants are either local or general, and act by increasing the vital power. Local stimuli either produce a determination of blood to the part, a secretion of semen, or the formation of pustules These substances are made into a paste and applied over the part. The general stimulants include carminatives, which stimulate the stomach and intestinal canal, and lead to the expulsion of flatulence. This numerous class of medicines have already been enumerated, under the head of aliments; which are used in powder or decoction, with, or without other medicines.

13. Astringents. There is a considerable list of astringents used for curing diarrhœa and dysentery, and of astringent tonics for the cure of ulcers, and for stopping hœmorrhage.

Among the anthelminitics, biringa viranga is the Embelia Ribes, and is still used as such in different parts of India.

14. Alteratives are medicines which

increase strength by removing diseased functions. It is only to adults and old people that this class of medicines is administered; and before giving it, an emetic or a purgative should be exhibited, as a cloth should first be cleaned before it is dried. There are four kinds of alteratives. The first promotes pleasures; the second cures diseases; the third increases memory and longvity; and the fourth prevents the usual changes of life, such as age, thirst, hunger, &c. 1. Cold water, milk, honey, and ghee may be taken internally, mixed or separately, to restore a proper degree of strength to the body. 2. Another kind of alteratives increases the memory, and lengthens the person's life. Various medicines are recommended for this purpose, and are powdered and mixed with sugar, kept in a vessel for seven days, and then used with cold water. During this treatment the person should reside in a close room, and continue the medicine for six months. He should only use rice, milk and sugar for food, and bathe in cold water towards evening. His memory will thus be improved, and he may live for a hundred years. This plan of treatment may be adopted in leprosy and dropsy, with the addition of cow's urine instead of water. With this medicine the juice of the mandukaparm (Hydrocotyle Asiaticc) is exhibited, after which milk should be taken, and barley, rice and ghee exhibited for three months.

3. Another kind retains the person young, prevents the hair turning grey and the teeth from falling out. If a man uses cold water, milk, honey, or ghee, separately or together, he will not soon have the marks of old age. For the same purpose other medicines are recommended.

15. Tonics, &c. The Sòma, sacred medicine, is said to produce longevity, and removes the marks of age. There are many fancied varieties of such medicines, unknown to the present sinful race of mankind. Numerous other drugs of this class are used for increasing the pleasure of the society of women; these are considered nutritions diet, as ghee and animal food, wholesome drink,

good news, anointing the body, especially towards the full moon, the presence of young women, love songs, clear nights, beautiful gardens, and a fine prospect ; also the use of betel-nut, wine, flowers, such as garlands round the neck, sweet smells, &c., are thought to have this effect. That powder of Vidara. (Flacourtia cataphracta),with ghee and honey, and also the powder of Amalaka (Phyllanthus smlica) mixed with sugar, honey, and ghee, the flour of barley, &c., with milk and the seeds of Atmagupta, (carpopgon pruriens) increase the person's happiness and desires. These will be diminished when bitter, hot, salt, or sour articles of food are eaten, which diminish the fluids. In like manner, desire will be removed by its abuse, by certain diseases of the external organs, and by the division of the vessels.

16. Oleaginous applications, such as oil, ghee, fat, &c., may be given by the mouth as food, as laxatives, as errhines, as enemata, as unguents, or as injections for the ear and urethra. There are two kinds, vegetable and animal oils. Of the latter cow's ghee is the

best, and the sesamum seed oil is the best of the vegetable variety. Some of this class of medicines are digested with difficulty, others with less difficulty, and a third kind easily. Ghee is good for weak persons who have a bad memory, or who are affected with poison, and diseases of wind and bile. Oil is to be used externally, but it may be given internally in cases of worms, and in costiveness. Warm water should be taken after the oleaginous substances.

17. Agents acting by depressing the vital powers are Refrigerants, such as cold infusions both internally and externally. Fire is also used.

18. Narcotics. Very few narcotics are mentioned in the ancient works; ganja or bhang, the resin of hemp, was used, and also datura. They likewise employed bish (aconitum ferox), kakola, (cocculus indicus); kaephul, (strychnos, nux vomica).

The Bujjerbhang of the Arabians, and the Dhumrapatra of the Hindus were, perhaps, the nicotiana tabacum of Linneus. According to the proclamation of the Emperor Jehangir mentioned in his memoirs, tobacco was introduced into India, either in his, or the preceding reign. It was discovered in Yucatan, a province in Mexico, in 1520 (Humboldt). Were not some of the varieties employed in Europe before this date.

18. Chemical Agents. These medicines are, 1st, Escharotics and caustics; 2nd, Lithontriptics, or solvents of urinary stone or gravel, are sometimes employed; for which purpose the usual diuretics are exhibited, particularly Arjuna, (Pentaptera Arjuna), and Ashwavedaka (Plectranthus scutellaroides, Roxb).

When administered by an ignorant person, medicine is a poison, and compared to the knife, fire, or lightning; but when administered with the necessary knowledge it is like the water of immortality. There are said to be two kinds of medicine, one of which gives strength to the body when no disease exists and the other arrests and cures diseases when they are present. In like manner poison may be administered in a proper manner, with great advantage in the cure of disease.

CHAPTER XVI.

HINDU HYGENE.

THE other nations of the world are of opinion that the Hindus are generally ignorant of the laws of health. How their notion is wrong will be conclusively proved by our giving, in the following pages, an account of the observations made by the ancient Hindu sages regarding Hygene or *Pathyapathya*. The Hindu legislators were convinced of the importance of the laws of health at a very early period and therefore they enacted various laws for the purpose. They combined these laws with their religion with the view that the people would implicity obey them and hence in our sacred books we find so many precepts regarding the laws of health. We have also a number of works on this subject not to speak of the Puranas every one of which contains lucid accounts of it.

They are rising from bed in the morning, cleaning the mouth and bathing, annointing the body, clothing, housing sleeping with use of exercise, food and drink. It is proper to rise from bed sometime before sun-rise, and after morning prayers, to perform the duties of nature with the face towards the north. The teeth should not be cleansed before the tenth year of the child's age; after which they are to be cleansed with a pice of a fresh branch of the neem. The mouth, eyes, and face are washed with water. The nails, beard and hair of the head are to be kept clean and trimmed every fifth day which promotes strength, longevity, purity and tranquility of mind.

Bathing.—The following are the most common kinds of bath: (1) the cold bath removes the impurities, inordinate heat and irritation of the surface, and retains the blood pure. The use of cold water strengthens vision, but in winter deranges phlegm and wind, and during the hot season warm bathing increases bile and blood. (2) Warm water-bath is generally prepared with medicinal plants and is used either generally or locally (3). Vapour baths are used for removing pain. They are made by heating a quanlity of water in an earthen pot over which a lid has been placed. The patient is first well rubbed with oil and then sits on a chair over a pot of water with a covering of clothes thrown over him. The Hindus are generally fond of rubbing oil. It has a effect over the system. It diminishes the deseases of wind and phlegm, increases the seven *dhâtu*, and improves the marrow, the color of the skin and the organs of sense. It cures deseases of the feet, prevents painful cramps of the fingers, and so long as the head is kept moistoured with oil it prevents headache, improves hair and prevents its becoming grey.

Clothing.—After bathing the body is to be well dried and rubbed. Silk and warm red clothes diminish the deseases of wind and phlegm and should be used in the winter season ; and clothing should be light, cool and thin during the hot weather. In rainy and cold weather warm clothes of a medium thickness are to be used.

Housing.—The ancient Hindus paid a very great attention to the building of houses with proper arrangements for ventelation. They are sufficiently raised to avoid damp and are religiously kept neat and clean.

Sleeping :—"Early to bed and early to rise" is one of the old and most approved maxims of the Hindus. They recommend sleeping on a large mat, in a comfortable house and at the accustomed time. Sleep keeps the humours in a healthy state, improves the colour of the skin, the health, appetite and strength. Sleeping during the day increases phlegm and fat and should be avoided by those in whom phlegm is increased during the spring, the rains and the winter months etc,. It may be indulged in the hot season.

Exercise.—Increases strength, prevents and cures desease by equalising the humours; it prevents fatness and laziness and increases the firmness of the body. Walking is always to be used by those persons who live on rich food. Evening and morning are the best times specially in the cold and spring months. Shampooing is also recommended by them.

Food.—The ancient Hindus paid very great attention to food. It gives strength and colour to the body; it supports the heat of the body, retains the humours in their just proportion, supports health and promotes longivity. Charaka divides food into stewed, boiled and hard food that requires to be chewed and liquid food. Sushruta arranges food into varieties of rice and corn, fruits, varieties of flesh, oils, flowers, fruits and herbs, salt and prepared food and drinks including water and various spirituous liquors. Various classes of food are thus arranged.

Sweet articles of food increase the milk and the fat while they improve the eyesight and relieve asthma, worms and affections of the throat. They also increase phlegm, the strength of the tissues, and the humours, retain the body in health and promote longevity.

Acid articles of food promote appetite, are cooling before and heating after eating. They promote digestion, and restore irregularities and derangements in the wind, bile and phlegm. They should not not be however taken often.

Salt articles of food relax the bowels, promote digestion and increase appetite. They also promote perspiration, remove derangement of the wind, and bile, phlegm and blood. If long continued they derange the humours.

Bitter food is not pleasant to taste, but is dry and light to the stomach, increases bile and air. It corrects too much bile and phlegm. But if always eaten it deranges the humours and produes deseases of wind.

Pungent articles of food are of a drying nature increasing the appitite and milk and diminishing thirst and fever. They cure diseases of phlegm but if taken too much they produce thirst, weakness and derange the spleen.

Astringent articles of food are cooling and cure deseases of the bile and phlegm.

But if taken for some time they produce costiveness.

Animal food and vegetables were also in great favour with the Early Hindus.

We will close this Chapter with speaking a few words on the use of water. They were very careful about their drinking water. They considered the water of wells or natural springs in the sandy beds of rivers as the most wholeseme as it promotes digestion and strength. The river and fountain water, at the bottom of the hills, was considered less wholesome, and the most unhealthy was the water from brooks and the stagnant water of tanks and reservoirs. This water was supposed to produce indigestion, obstructions, lethargy, with a predisposition to fever.

CHAPTER XVII.

HINDU SURGERY.

Susruta considered surgery as the branch of medicine most esteemed as it had reached a high state of perfection at an early period. The importance of surgeons, possessing a knowledge of anatomy, with the nature and relative position of parts, to enable them to perform operation, was well-known to the ancient Hindus. According to the Hindus surgery considers the cure of external deseases by the hand, by instruments or by topical applications. The accidents, which must have frequently occured among a race of people given to hunting and agriculture and; the feuds that were so frequent among small states, induced the Hindu sages, at an early period, to attend to surgical deseases. This led them to believe that surgery had been the branch of medicine first cultivated and explains the importance in which the ancient writers held this branch of the healing art, the attention which they bestowed upon it and the ability with which they exercised it. The ancient Hindu practitioners were bold and expert surgeons accustomed to perform cystotomy, lithotomy, embryotomy, autoplastic operations, couching for cataract, paracentesis thoracis and abdominis &c.

The sages explain the early age at which surgery was practised by the necessity of curing the wounds inflicted in the battles of the gods. The two Aswinis performed many wonderful surgical feats. Surgery forms the first chapter of Susruta and in the Ayur-Veda it is considered to form the first two of the eight departments of the medical science and Dhanwantari was born to teach this and other departments of the medical Science. The early Hindu medical practitioners also used a number of surgical instruments. This great variety of instruments shows how carefully they studied surgery. The hand is always represented as the first, the best, and the most important of all surgical instruments as it is with its assistance that all operations are performed. The surgical instruments should be made of the best iron reduced to steel a process early known to the Hindus. They are generally six inches in length of which the blade forms the half or quarter. They should have good handles and firm joints, be well polished and sufficintly sharp to divide a hair; they should be quite clean, wrapped in flannel and kept in a wooden box. There are twenty ancient cutting instruments mentioned by Susruta. There are one hundred and one blunt instruments such as curved or hooked instruments to remove teeth and splinters of bones or foreign bodies. They are usually of iron, eighteen finger-breadths long, having heads shaped like those of animals, the beaks of birds etc: a smaller kind will remove foreign substances lodged in the ear, nose etc. There are twenty varieties of tubular instruments of different sizes and shapes including catheters, syringes etc. They are used for removing obstructions or substances from deep seated canals as the intestines, urethra &c., for examining deep seated parts and for drawing off fluids, etc. There are twenty-eight kinds of probes, rods and sounds varying in size and shape for examing the size and nature of foreign objects lodged in parts of difficult access, and for clearing canals particularly the urethra. Some of these are rounded like a half-pea or the earth, worm or the point of an arrow; and another has a hand like the foot-staff of a cylindrical form like the malectee flower and is often used in clearing the uretha. Some of these probes have small cavities at their extremeties for applying caustics etc., to the diseased part: very much the same form as is now used for strictures and in some diseases of the vagina and uterus. Some rods have extremeties like the rose-apple and are curved; these are to be applied heated. A variety of forceps with claws, resembling the half of the stone of the plum, are for eradicating polypi, a frequent and troublesome disease in Hindustan; which is relieved by forcibly extracting irritable excrescence. Other accessory instruments are enumerated as thread-bandages, leaves, leather, bark, silk cloth, loadstone, pins and tents. The finger-nails, tongue, teeth etc. were also employed.

The early ancient Hindu teachers used to deliver to their pupils practical instructions for surgical operations. After the student has been taught the science of healing by books he was next instructed in the use of instrumentals. Without practical skill theoretical knowledge was considered of no use. The different surgical operations were shown to the student upon wax spread out upon a board, on gourds, cucumbers and other soft fruits; tapping and puncturing was practised on a leather bag of water or soft mud; sacrification and bleeding was practised upon the fresh bodies of animals from which the hair has been removed as upon dead bodies; and puncturing or lancing on the hollow stalks of water lilies or the vessels of dead animals. Dexterity was thus acquired before exercising it on human body. The manner of holding the knife and using the probe was practised upon a piece of hollow bamboo or the like; the removal of substances from cavities by removing the large seeds of the jack fruit or bel fruit. The extraction of teeth was practised upon dead bodies and animals. Sewing was practised upon leather and cloth. The application of bandages and ligatures was exercised upon flexible models of the human body; the means of making noses, ears etc., was practised upon dead animals; and the application of caustics and cauteries on animals. The use of injection was exercised with a water-pot having a tube passing into it.

There are eight kinds of surgical operations: incision as in fistula-in-ans; opening parts as of large abscesses or drawing lines, by which the parts are sacrificed or inoculated; puncturing as in opening veins in hydrocele and in dropsy; probing or sounding parts, as in fistula to ascertain the presence of foreign substances; the operation of extraction, as of the stone, of the teeth and of the fœtus; removal of fluids as pus, blood etc., or of bad humours as in leprous blotches, in elephantisis; and sewing parts together with thread or twine or small ligatures made of the skin of animals or fibures of vegetable substances, roots, hair etc., as in wound specially near joints.

When an operation is decided on a fortunate moment is selected. A clean and well-lighted room is to be chosen in which the operation is to be performed ; and bandages, the leaves of trees, thread, honey, ghee, the juices of different kinds of trees, milk, oil, cold and hot water are to be in readiness and strong and steady assistants to hold the patient while care is taken not to frighten him. The patient is to be placed with his face to the east and the surgeon before him with his face to the west.

The knife should be wet with water before being used. The season for operating is when the sky is clear in the rains and during the evenings and mornings in the hot weather. If possible, operations should be performed near the new moon, as this is the most favourable time. If the person is weak, much diseased or insensible, or if the disease has come on suddenly the operation should be performed during the evening or morning when the weather is steady and seasonable.

When a boil is to be opened or the flesh divided the part is first to have certain escharotics rubbed over it to diminish the pain. When a vessel, joint or sensible part is to be divided oil is first to be rubbed over it. The surgeon should hold the knife firm in the hand; if it has been thurst into a boil and no pus follows it is to be quickly withdrawn. If then be much pus it may be opened several times when necessary. The surgeon should be strong and operate quickly; his knife should be good and he should neither perspire, shake, nor make exclamations. In performing operations the sensible parts of the body are to be avoided: as the palms of the hands and soles of the feet, vessels, tendons, joints and bones. When near vital organs the knife should be held so as to cut outwards; and should any such organ be wounded it produces severe pain and is cured with difficulty. If the vital part in an extremity is wounded, it is to be amputated to save the individual's life. If the bone of the head or breast be broken, it is to be raised by the assistance of the instruments:

When the foetus is dead in the uterus in ascitis, piles or in certain excrescences and swellings near the anus which have existed upwards of a month the patient is to take dinner before the operation and it is to be completed while withdrawing the knife ; cold water is then to be applied to the part, the pus is to be squeezed and part cleansed with tepid water. Lint smeared with honey or ghee is then to be put into the wound to prevent its closing. The wound is to be rubbed with honey or ghee and a bandage is then to be placed round the part.

Graphic accounts of various important operations are given in Sushruta. Here we will give two to show our readers how minute and careful the Hindu surgeons were. The first is *lithotomy*. Gravel and stone are very common in some parts of Hindustan. The calculi, from the more relaxed state and less nervous temparament of the person, pass more easily with the urine than in more temperate climates; and are often found implanted near the extremity of the urethra and require to be removed by enlarging the

the orifice, or when at a distance from the extremity by cutting down the calculus.

The Hindu writers suppose that a urinary calculus is produced by deranged humours and the physician is recommended to restore these derangements and to cure the disease. But when this is not accomplished it is necessary to have recourse to the knife; when the operation is decided on the patient must have aparients and ghee administered internally for several days previous to the operation. When robust the strength of the patient is to be reduced in the usual way. Before the operation the instruments should be arranged so as to be at hand when required. He is to be placed on a table, supported by a person behind who separates his legs which are to be bent and tied to the two wrists. The abdomen is then to be rubbed downwards so as to make the stone descend; while the index and middle fingers of the left-hand, well-oiled, are introduced into the rectum and the stone felt and brought low in the pirineum, so as to make a protuberance should the patient faint at this stage of the operation, it should not be proceeded with, else the patient will die. An incision is then to be made over the stone, on the left side of the perineum, a barley-corn in breadth from the raphe, and an inch from the anus, and carried down to the stone. The incision is then to be enlarged in proportion to the size of the stone, and it is removed by an iron scoop. If there be more than one stone they must all be removed, taking care not to break the stone, nor to leave any fragments behind, as it will, in such a case, slowly form again. These small fragments may be removed by scoop.

The incision may be made on the right side of the perineum, always taking care during the operation to avoid the raphe with the seminal canals, the vessels of the spermatic cord and the rectum. If the seminal canals or the spermatic vessels are wounded, the person will become impotent.

After the stone has been removed, place the patient in a hip-bath of warm water to promote perspiration, and to prevent the accumulation of blood in the bladder. Should this collection of blood take place it is to be removed by injecting a decoction of the Ficus Indica by means of a syringe. To heal the urinary passages, administer sherbets, and apply honey and ghee to the wound. Barley-water with warm ghee is to be given twice or thrice a day, for three days, to keep the urine pure, and then give sugar, rice and milk in small quantities for ten days; and fruits, and broths made of the flesh of game animals for ten days; and for ten more days, promote perspiration by means of warm fomentations with oil and ghee.

When the calculus is small and produced by semen and cannot be disloged from the urethera by pressure, an incision is to be made over it, and the calculus removed, by means of a hook.

After the operation of lithotomy, riding on horse-back, or elephants, or carriages, as well as venery, should be avoided for a year. The patient should also avoid swimming in water so as to stretch the wound too much, and eating indigestible food to irritate it.

Next we will give an account of how a

nose is to be restored. When such a deformity is to be restored, a fresh leaf is cut of exactly the size of the nose, it is then to be placed upon the cheek, and the necessary quantity of skin and cellular membrane is to be traced. The remains of the nose are then scarified, and after dissecting up the flap, it is to be placed upon the raw part of the nose, to which it will adhere. Sutures and bandages are applied to keep the parts together. After the bandage has been applied, a couple of wooden canulæ are to be introduced into the nostril to allow breathing, and to support the new nose. A piece of linen cloth previously soaked in oil is to be applied over the bandage. An aperient is then to be given to the patient, and his general health is to be attended to.

What we have given before will give our readers an idea of the skill and care of the early Hindu surgeons. They have left for us also an account of surgical accidents, as fractures, dislocations, etc., and how they are to be treated.

THE END.